History of Rheumatology

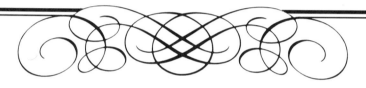

Charley J. Smyth, M.D.

Richard H. Freyberg, M.D.

Currier McEwen, M.D.

Arthritis Foundation
Atlanta, Georgia

Library of Congress Cataloging in Publication Data

Smyth, Charley J., 1909-
    History of rheumatology.

    Bibliography: p.
    Includes index.
    1. Rheumatism—United States—History.
2. Rheumatism—United States—Societies, etc.—
History.   I. Freyberg, Richard H., 1904-
II. McEwen, Currier.   III. Title.
RC927.S63   1985   362.1'96722   85-6197
ISBN 0-912423-01-3

Staff: Ann B. McGuire, Managing Editor
        Sharon E. Russell, Assistant Editor

Arthritis Foundation catalog number 3034   ISBN 0-912423-01-3

Contents

To Floyd B. Odlum, Chairman of the Board of Directors of the Arthritis Foundation, 1948 to 1970, Honorary Member of the American Rheumatism Association, respected by the medical profession and arthritis health professionals for his dedication to the cause of rheumatism, a man to whom all patients with arthritis are in debt, and a great friend of the authors, this book is dedicated.

Opposite: Portrait of Floyd B. Odlum painted in 1955 by President Dwight D. Eisenhower

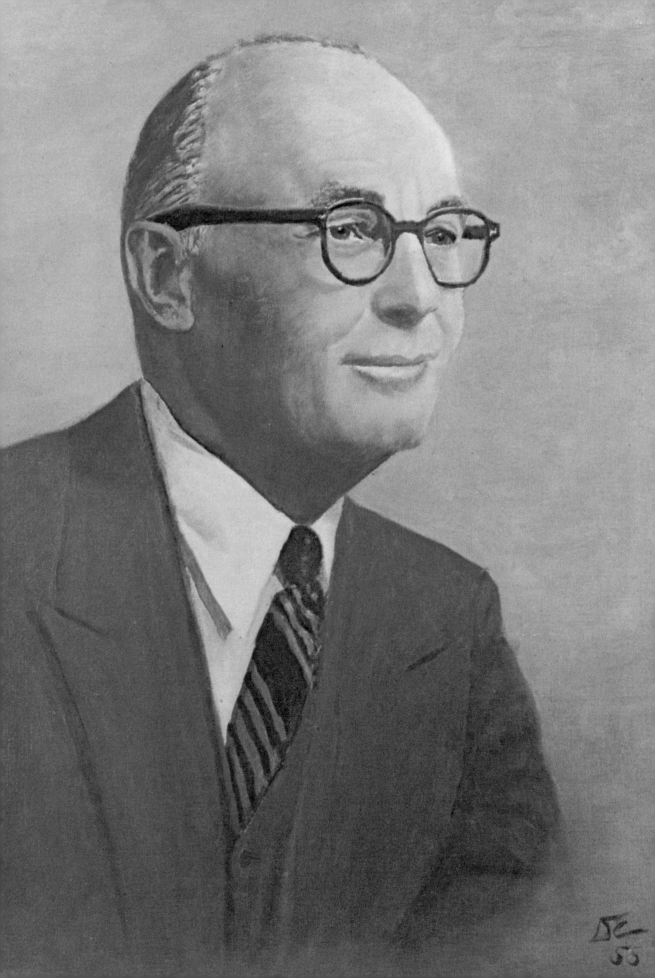

Preface

Progress in the rheumatic diseases during the present century has paralleled, if not exceeded, that in most other areas of medicine. The development of this branch of medicine in the United States represents but a segment of the worldwide history of arthritis. Rheumatology in this country had its origins in several lands, and the pioneers who advanced its development were trained in Europe and introduced methods of treatment and teaching based on European models. Dr. Ralph Pemberton of Philadelphia, Dr. Robert Osgood of Boston, and Dr. Philip Hench of the Mayo Clinic were prominent early leaders who promoted arthritis in America similar to the manner developed in Europe by Professor Jan van Breemen of Amsterdam.

While the dependence of American rheumatology on the developments in Europe is clear, it seemed desirable to present a comprehensive picture of the contributions of Americans, particularly in light of the rapid progress made in the United States in the past 50 years. This book is an outgrowth of discussions among the three authors and the encouragement of others to assemble the background information and describe the events that led to the establishment of this subspecialty of medicine. It is hoped that this historical review will be of interest to those in the medical and allied health professions, particularly the teachers, investigators, physical and occupational therapists, orthopedic and hand surgeons, and physicians treating patients with arthritis, and to lay men and women interested in arthritis. Also, we hope it serves as a stimulus to undergraduate and graduate students, residents, and fellows who have chosen rheumatology as a career.

Our presentation of this material is devoted in large part to a record of individuals who made significant contributions and the organizations that have had roles in the development of this subspecialty of medicine. Since the rapid growth and high level of achievement can be attributed largely to the stimulation and continued leadership of professional, philanthropic, and governmental organizations, separate consideration has been given to each of these groups. Much of the progress in rheumatology can be attributed to individual members of the American Rheumatism Association. The founding, rapid progress, and continuous support of the Arthritis and Rheumatism Foundation (now Arthritis Foundation) have played a major role in the history. Also, the commitment and sustained funding by the federal government through the National Institutes of Health have made possible many of the advances in arthritis research and training.

In preparing this review, we have attempted to record the significant contributions and identify those persons and organizations responsible. However, it is likely that some have been given inadequate or no consideration. An apology for this oversight is freely made, with confidence that the reader and those intimately concerned with current rheumatologic activities will recognize that omissions are inevitable in an effort of this magnitude.

Preface

In the last chapter, the authors, based upon their lifetime experiences in rheumatic diseases, present an historical account of the most important contributions toward a better understanding of the rheumatic diseases and improvement in the treatment of patients with arthritis. Included are many of the mistakes in therapy made over the years.

The authors wish to acknowledge the invaluable assistance given by our many colleagues who provided photographs, historical documents, and records. Through the help of Dr. Allen R. Myers, Chairman of the General Publications Committee of the American Rheumatism Association, the generous assistance was obtained of a distinguished panel of authorities to review particular sections of this book. Those who served were: Dr. J. Claude Bennett, Birmingham; Dr. William S. Clark, New York; Dr. John L. Decker, Bethesda; Dr. Joseph L. Hollander, Philadelphia; Dr. Ronald W. Lamont-Havers, Boston; Dr. Howard F. Polley, Bloomington, Indiana; Dr. William D. Robinson, Ann Arbor, Michigan; Mr. W. W. Satterfield, Little Rock; Dr. Charles L. Short, Boston; Dr. J. Sidney Stillman, Middleton, Rhode Island; Mr. H M Poole, Jr., La Jolla, California; and Dr. Emmerson Ward, Port Ludlow, Washington. Special recognition is given to Ms. Gail K. Riggs, M.A. for her invaluable assistance in preparing the history of the Arthritis Health Professions Association. Also, we are deeply indebted to Dr. Frederic C. McDuffie, Senior Vice President for Medical Affairs of the Arthritis Foundation, and Ms. Ann B. McGuire, Managing Editor of Professional Publications of the Arthritis Foundation, and her staff for their advice and guidance.

Grateful appreciation is expressed to Merck Sharp & Dohme, who have given encouragement and generous financial support to the Arthritis Foundation to make this publication possible.

Charley J. Smyth, M.D.
Richard F. Freyberg, M.D.
Currier McEwen, M.D.

About the Authors

Charley J. Smyth received his undergraduate education at the University of Michigan and his MD degree from Jefferson Medical College of Philadelphia. He served on the house staff in medicine, received a masters degree in pathology, and was a physician at the University of Michigan Hospital from 1935-42, joining the new Rackham Arthritis Research Unit in 1937. During World War II he was Medical Director at the Wayne County General Hospital and taught at Wayne State University in Detroit.

Dr. Smyth moved west to accept an appointment at the Medical School of the University of Colorado as Director of Post Graduate Education and subsequently served on that faculty as Professor of Medicine and Head of the Division of Rheumatic Diseases for more than 25 years. After retiring from this administrative position, he became the first Medical Director of the newly established Alpert Arthritis Treatment Center at Denver's Rose Medical Center and remained as Clinical Professor at the University of Colorado. During these years, he was a consultant on the staffs of many Denver hospitals, including the Fitzsimons Army Hospital and the Denver Veterans Administration Hospital.

He is the author of more than 100 scientific articles and contributions to textbooks on subjects relating to the diagnosis and evaluation of therapy of various types of arthritis; he served as editor of four biannual issues of the *Rheumatism Reviews*. His contributions to national medical organizations include serving as President of the American Rheumatism Association and the National Society of Clinical Rheumatologists and as a Trustee of the American Society of Internal Medicine, and representing Colorado as Governor of the American College of Physicians. He was a founding member of the Arthritis Foundation and assisted in the establishment of the Michigan and Colorado chapters and served as President of the latter.

Richard H. Freyberg was born and raised in Goshen, Indiana. After receiving his undergraduate degree from the University of Michigan in 1926, he entered the Michigan Medical School, graduating in 1930. After internship and residency training in internal medicine at the University of Michigan Hospital, he was appointed Instructor and later Assistant Professor of Medicine at the Michigan Medical School. In 1937 he was chosen to establish the Rackham Arthritis Research Unit at this institution and directed its research program until 1944. That year, he moved to New York City to become Director of the newly established Division of Rheumatic Diseases at The Hospital for Special Surgery, Chief of the Arthritis Clinic at New York Hospital, and Associate Clinical Professor (later Clinical Professor) of Medicine at Cornell University Medical College.

Throughout his professional career, Dr. Freyberg was actively engaged in investigation of the major forms of rheumatism, with particular interest in pathogenesis, therapy, clinical management of patients, and training of developing rheumatologists.

He was active in the American Rheumatism Association soon after its formation; he was President in 1948-49. He served as President of the New York Rheumatism Association in 1958. Dr. Freyberg was a founder of the Arthritis Foundation, a director for 22 years, and recipient of its Floyd B. Odlum Award in 1962. He served on the first National Arthritis and Metabolic Disease Council from 1949-52 and held a second term from 1955-57. He was President of the Pan-American League Against Rheumatism from 1953-57.

His membership in medical societies includes: American College of Physicians (Master), American Society of Clinical Investigation, Central Society for Clinical Research, New York Academy of Medicine, Harvey Society, and numerous foreign national rheumatism societies (honorary).

Currier McEwen was born in Newark, New Jersey in 1902, the son of a physician severely crippled by psoriatic arthritis. He attended Newark Academy and Wesleyan University and received the MD degree from New York University in 1926. After internship and residency at Bellevue Hospital, he spent four years in research on rheumatic fever with Dr. Homer F. Swift at the Rockefeller Institute (now Rockefeller University) before returning to NYU School of Medicine in 1932 as Instructor in Medicine and Assistant Dean. He was Dean from 1937-55. In 1932 he started the NYU Study Group on Rheumatic Diseases and served as its chairman until 1968. In 1970 he retired as Professor Emeritus of Medicine.

Dr. McEwen became a member of the American Rheumatism Association in 1934 and was President in 1952-53. He was active in the formation of the Arthritis Foundation and was a member of the Medical and Scientific Committee 1948-62 (chairman 1953-57), a member of the Board of Directors 1953-57, and Chairman of the Board of the New York Chapter in 1958. He was active also in the affairs of the National Institute of Arthritis and Metabolic Diseases, serving as a member of the National Advisory Council from 1954-58 and Chairman of its Program-Project Committee from 1960-62.

His other medical society memberships include the American Society of Clinical Investigation, Association of American Physicians, Interurban Clinical Club, American College of Physicians (Master), New York Academy of Medicine, Harvey Society, and honorary membership in foreign rheumatism societies. He has honorary doctorates of science from Wesleyan University and Marietta College.

Dr. McEwen entered World War II as Executive Officer of the First General Hospital (Bellevue Hospital–affiliated unit) and subsequently was Medical Consultant, Brittany Base Section; Commanding Officer, 49th Station Hospital in England; and Chief Consultant in Medicine, European Theater, with rank of colonel.

He is author or coauthor of some 190 articles and chapters on rheumatic diseases. He has four children and six grandchildren. He and his wife Elisabeth now live in South Harpswell, Maine, where he continues a part-time rheumatologic consulting practice, is active with the Maine Chapter of AF, writes, and hybridizes irises. As both an irisologist and a rheumatologist, Dr. McEwen found a unique indication for colchicine; he used this gout-relieving drug to induce tetraploidy in normally diploid Siberian and Japanese irises, resulting in irises with larger flowers and more pronounced features. He has received seven annual awards from the American Iris Society for his beautiful irises.

1

The Early Twentieth Century

The Dismal Years and the Transition to the Modern Period

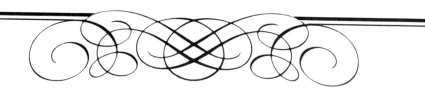

THROUGHOUT the colonial period and the years of western expansion in the United States, the care of the sick was largely in the hands of physicians educated in Europe or trained in this country in a manner resembling apprenticeship. By the mid-1800s the developing United States medical schools were the major source of physicians and also provided centers of intellectual stimulation and research. To be sure, research was all too limited by lack of funds to support scientifically skilled full-time investigators, but the practice of medicine was influenced most beneficially. One result was the appearance of physicians with special interests in particular branches of medicine, and specialization became a very positive trend. The physician whose main concern was tuberculosis was an early example of this trend, as were those with primary interest in nutrition, cardiology, and other aspects of internal medicine. Unfortunately, treatment continued to be largely empiric and symptomatic and, for the most part, of limited effectiveness. Nevertheless, important steps were made in the understanding of various diseases and in the differentiation of one from another. Therapy, although inadequate, began to be more rational and critically evaluated in most branches of medicine.

Unfortunately, this was not true for what many years later became known as rheumatology. One of the most important advances of the late 1800s was the development of the science of bacteriology. This, of course, launched a new era of scientific advances in the understanding and treatment of infectious diseases, but led to an erroneous theory that dominated arthritis treatment for some 30 years and was the most significant reason that the early decades of the twentieth century saw rheumatology at its lowest point.

Between 1910 and 1920, the idea that foci of infection were the cause of arthritis, a theory originally proposed by Dr. Benjamin Rush in 1805, was revived by Dr. Frank Billings (13). Rush had reported a patient with arthritis whose cure he attributed to extraction of a diseased tooth (132). Billings, a respected professor at the Rush Medical

College in Chicago and influential in the American Medical Association, expanded Rush's theory to include focal infection not only in the teeth but also in the tonsils, gall bladder, and other organs more easily removable in the early twentieth century than in the nineteenth. Billings' ideas were almost universally accepted, both in the United States and Europe, and dominated medical thinking into the 1930s. Extirpation of these suspected foci was usually the first step in the treatment of patients with arthritis. Vast numbers of innocent teeth, tonsils, gall bladders, and other organs were removed because of this theory.

A logical, though equally inappropriate and ineffective, further development of this theory was the use of vaccines prepared from bacteria grown from suspected foci. Usually "stock" vaccines provided by commercial laboratories from cultures of staphylococci, diphtheroids, and other bacteria were used, but physicians specializing in the treatment of arthritis often prepared so-called autogenous vaccines from bacteria isolated from the individual patients.

Along with removal of foci and injection of vaccines was the practice of high colonic irrigations to "rid the body of toxic wastes." These treatments were so popular that commercially operated "parlors" for giving such lavages flourished throughout the country at that time.

It is not surprising that many internists and others on the staffs of medical schools could not accept these concepts and measures of treatment. As Dr. Robert M. Stecher said, "In 1925 dignified physicians looked with suspicion on the band of technicians, Swedish masseurs, medicinal hydrologists, other dedicated enthusiasts and pseudoquacks who bothered themselves with the lame and the halt" (140). The specialty of what is now rheumatology was in those early decades of the twentieth century scarcely academically respectable. Teaching in medical schools included instruction in rheumatic fever, chiefly because of its prevalence in children and its importance as a cause of heart disease. Gout also received attention. Tuberculous and gonococcal arthritis and Charcot's joints were considered briefly in lectures on the underlying diseases, but the most important and common forms of arthritis received little or no mention. This disinterest stemmed in part from the sad lack of knowledge, but also from dissatisfaction with the prevailing treatments.

Aside from studies on rheumatic fever, research was scant. Funding for research in general was limited at that time, and then as now, money for scientific studies went mainly to those concerned with life-threatening diseases. Nevertheless, some significant work was done. Of particular importance were the studies of pathology of joint structures by Drs. Edward H. Nichols and Frank L. Richardson in 1909 that clearly distinguished the lesions of rheumatoid arthritis from those of degenerative arthritis (98).

Confusion regarding rheumatic diseases was compounded by the fact that a standard nomenclature was lacking. Often a term in a medical journal might mean different diseases to the author and the reader. Despite the findings of Nichols and Richardson, the differences between rheumatoid and degenerative arthritis were not appreciated by most physicians, with the result that vaccines and removal of suspected foci were used even for the treatment of degenerative joint disease.

The situation in hospitals was deplorable. The lack of interest in chronic diseases— except for tuberculosis in the special institutions devoted to that illness—and the desire to have beds for the acutely ill patients led to the practice of getting rid of patients crippled by arthritis as quickly as possible. One of the first orders written after admission of a patient with a chronic form of arthritis in a general hospital was likely to be to arrange for transfer to a chronic disease hospital. Unfortunately, interest in and treatment of these patients in such institutions were, with few exceptions, rarely better than the care they received in the general hospitals.

Fortunately, a few physicians did show a special interest in chronic arthritis. For some this interest resulted from concern about relatives with severe crippling. In others it stemmed primarily from an urge to care for patients who were so in need of help and to study diseases for which knowledge was so abysmal. One must approach the responsibility of mentioning these "pioneers" with considerable trepidation because of the certainty of omitting some who should be named. In the remainder of this chapter, individuals and institutions with special concern for the care of arthritis patients during the first four decades of the twentieth century are presented on a roughly geographic and chronologic basis. The important rheumatologic units that marked the beginning of the modern period—the Mayo Clinic, Harvard University, Columbia University, New York University, University of Michigan, and University of Pennsylvania—are discussed in more detail in the following chapter. In the discussion of institutions, the stories are continued briefly beyond the 1940 endpoint of these two chapters to allow mention of those who carried the programs at those institutions forward.

PIONEERS

Philadelphia. Among the earliest physicians with particular interest in arthritis was Dr. Ralph Pemberton, who is often considered the father of rheumatology in the United States. His interest in arthritis had been stimulated during World War I when he had the opportunity to study many soldiers with arthritis. He was probably the first person in this country to attempt to define a physiologic or biochemical abnormality characteristic of chronic arthritis (107). Dr. Pemberton also was one of the first in this country to limit his practice to rheumatology, and he started the first arthritis clinic in Pennsylvania in 1926 at the Presbyterian Hospital. A few years later, he moved to the Abingdon Memorial Hospital. His leading role in the organization of the American Committee for the Study and Control of Rheumatism and, subsequently, the American Rheumatism Association (ARA) is discussed in Chapter 3. He served as chairman of the American Committee at its formation in 1926 and was president of the American Rheumatism Association in 1938–39. Dr. Pemberton was also the first American president of the International League Against Rheumatism, serving through the World War II years.

Also in Philadelphia, Dr. John Lansbury started an arthritis clinic for teaching as well as care of patients at Temple University Hospital in 1938. The contributions of Drs. Comroe, Hollander, and others of that city are discussed in Chapter 2.

Baltimore. That great clinician, Dr. William Osler, during his years as Professor of Medicine at Johns Hopkins University directed his extraordinary acumen and insight into many rheumatologic problems. Of particular importance were a series of three articles written between 1895 and 1903 on what today is called systemic lupus erythematosus (100–102). More than 50 years before a laboratory test was devised to aid in the diagnosis of that disease, Dr. Osler had identified and described a group of patients, most of whom can be accepted today as having various manifestations of systemic lupus. Drs. Tumulty and Harvey (155) noted that Osler first emphasized the fundamental concept that the alterations occurring in the skin of patients with systemic lupus had their counterpart in the internal organs and that systemic manifestations can occur in the absence of dermal abnormalities. Dr. Osler also noted that the endocardium was sometimes involved, antedating by some 30 years the findings of Libman and Sacks (78). He realized the kinship of the rheumatic diseases but also the possibility of different causes.

Dr. Maxwell Lockie came to the Johns Hopkins Hospital in September 1931 as an assistant resident at the Marburg Medical Service and was given permission to start an arthritis clinic. The clinic, which met five days weekly with the assistance of the orthopedic staff, began in December 1931 as part of the orthopedic clinic (79). Dr. Lockie left the following year to return to Buffalo. Dr. Charles Wainwright, a member of the Department of Medicine, began a weekly arthritis clinic in 1932. It was not until 1955, however, that the outstanding Connective Tissue Division was established under the direction of Dr. Lawrence E. Shulman, as a subdivision of the Department of Medicine. From the start, the potential of this unit was apparent, and it was awarded one of the first research training grants made by the National Institute of Arthritis and Metabolic Diseases. Dr. Shulman served as director until he moved to the National Institute of Arthritis, Diabetes and Digestive and Kidney Diseases (NIADDK) (see Chapter 10) in 1976, when his place was taken by Dr. Mary Betty Stevens.

New York. In New York, as elsewhere in the United States in the mid-1800s, interest in the treatment of arthritis was found primarily among orthopedists. Dr. Lewis Sayre, Professor of Orthopedic Surgery at the Bellevue Hospital Medical College and the first professor of orthopedics in this country, carried on his pioneering surgical and nonsurgical measures for arthritis at Bellevue Hospital.

Dr. James A. Knight was another orthopedist who became dedicated to helping the many patients with crippling and deformities in this rapidly growing city of 800,000. He was adept at the construction and use of braces for lame patients and trusses for those with hernias. With the help of Mr. Robert Hartley, secretary of the Association for the Improvement of the Condition of the Poor, funds were obtained and the Society for the Relief of the Ruptured and Crippled was incorporated in 1863. A hospital of 28 beds was established in Dr. Knight's home. The hospital prospered and in 1870 moved to a 200-bed facility. Subsequently, Dr. Virgil P. Gibney and other outstanding orthopedists and general surgeons led the hospital, which later became increasingly concerned with the orthopedic management of crippling from arthritis. In 1924 an arthritis clinic was started under the direction of Dr. R. Garfield Snyder, who was joined by Drs. Cornelius Traeger and William Squires, both active in the New York Rheumatism Association and the Arthritis Foundation. In 1939 the name of the hospital was changed to The Hospital for Special Surgery. In 1944 Dr. Richard Freyberg left his post as Director of the Rheumatology Program at the University of Michigan to become physician-in-chief. Research on various rheumatologic problems expanded under his direction as did undergraduate and graduate medical education.

Subsequently, the hospital became affiliated with the New York Hospital–Cornell Medical Center and moved once more in 1955 to become a part of that complex of medical and nursing schools, hospitals, and research units. With the leadership of Dr. Freyberg and later Dr. Charles L. Christian as physicians-in-chief and Dr. Philip D. Wilson as surgeon-in-chief, the hospital continued to grow in importance as a center for rheumatologic care, teaching, and research.

Probably the first New Yorker who could be considered a rheumatologist, in the sense of devoting his practice solely to rheumatic diseases, was Dr. Reginald Burbank. His interest in arthritis led to the founding of an arthritis clinic at the Cornell Clinic in New York City in 1915. The following year he moved across First Avenue to Bellevue Hospital Medical College as instructor in orthopedic surgery under Dr. Reginald Sayre and became chief of an arthritis clinic at Bellevue Hospital from 1917 to 1926. Influenced by the views of Dr. Billings, he and a bacteriologist, L. G. Hadjopoulos, undertook bacteriologic studies that convinced them a streptococcus caused rheumatoid arthritis. They believed the intestinal tract was the source of the infection and hence were less insistent on the then-current measure of removing teeth, tonsils, and other suspected foci. Dr. Burbank was an ardent believer in the value of vaccines prepared from streptococci isolated from the individual patient but also made good use of rest, salicylates, physical therapy, and orthopedic measures to help his patients. In 1928 he founded the American Society for the Study of Arthritis, which existed for 12 years or more, but that group did not later merge with the American Rheumatism Association, and Dr. Burbank was never a member of the latter.

Among the most influential rheumatologists of this early period in New York was Dr. Russell LaFayette Cecil. Born in Kentucky in 1881, he attended Princeton and the Medical College of Virginia and had housestaff experience at the Johns Hopkins Hospital before moving to New York. In the Department of Pathology at Columbia University Presbyterian Hospital Medical Center, he worked with Drs. Warfield Loncope and Homer Swift attempting to induce lesions of rheumatic fever in rabbits by the injection of streptococci. These efforts failed, but rheumatology and streptococci became major interests for him. When World War I broke out, Dr. Cecil entered the army in 1917 as Director of Laboratories at Camp Upton. Pneumonia, a catastrophic military problem, especially during the influenza epidemic of 1918 to 1920, preempted his attention. His clinical and laboratory studies of the patients at Camp Upton led to his appointment as head of the Surgeon General's commission to study pneumonia.

After the war, he returned to New York and a faculty position at the Cornell University Medical College. At that time his practice was chiefly concerned with pneumonia; arthritis was a second interest, undoubtedly stimulated by his mother's severe rheumatoid arthritis. Although Dr. Cecil had made important bacteriologic contributions in the treatment of pneumonia, particularly in the use of vaccines and antisera, the advent of antibiotics made it clear that a far more efficacious treatment was at hand that would not require specialists and he turned his major attention to arthritis.

He was appointed chief of the arthritis clinic at the Cornell Clinic in 1922 and developed rheumatology rounds at the Cornell Division of Bellevue Hospital, where he also established a laboratory for bacteriologic research. Although at first a staunch advocate of the theory of focal infection as the cause of rheumatoid arthritis, he was subsequently influential in its discard.

No account of Dr. Cecil can fail to mention his monumental contribution as editor of the textbook known by all as "Cecil's Medicine." The first edition appeared in 1927 and was followed by many others; it replaced Osler's *Principles and Practice of Medicine* as the leading text in internal medicine. Dr. Cecil was also important in organizing rheumatology in the United States. His role in the development of the American Rheumatism Association and the Arthritis Foundation is discussed in other chapters. He was President of the American Association for the Study and Control of Rheumatic Diseases in 1936–37.

Also in New York, Dr. Otto Steinbrocker became concerned with arthritis because of his mother's severe crippling while he was an undergraduate at New York University School of Medicine in 1927. After a vain search for a place where he could obtain training in rheumatology, he was encouraged by Dr. Harlow Brooks to start an arthritis section on Brooks' service at City Hospital. Subsequently, in 1932, he established an arthritis clinic on the Fourth Division of Bellevue Hospital. An indefatigable worker, he was also author of a text on arthritis and chairman of the ARA committee to establish standards to guide the treatment of rheumatoid arthritis (142). He was President of ARA in 1950–51.

Also at that time, Dr. Walter Gay Lough, head of the Department of Medicine at the New York Post-Graduate Medical School and Hospital, encouraged Dr. Edward F. Hartung to establish an arthritis clinic at the hospital in 1924. A particular strength of that unit was Dr. Robert L. Preston, one of the first of the New York orthopedists to have primary interest in arthritis. Dr. Hartung was seriously involved in postgraduate teaching and subsequently made significant contributions to the development of postgraduate teaching in rheumatology at New York University when the Post-Graduate Medical School and Hospital merged with the New York University Medical Center. He also had important roles in organizational aspects of rheumatology. He was a member of the American Association for the Study and Control of Rheumatic Diseases and a founding member of the ARA. He served on various committees of the ARA and was its Secretary-Treasurer from 1955 to 1959 and President in 1960–61.

Dr. William B. Rawls was another New York physician of the 1930s whose major interest was the rheumatic diseases and who was active in the affairs of the New York Rheumatism Association and the New York Chapter of the Arthritis Foundation.

Boston. In Boston, too, the story of arthritis in the 1800s and early 1900s is that of orthopedic surgery. Dr. John Ball Brown practiced orthopedic surgery at the Massachusetts General Hospital from 1817 to 1833, when he established the Boston Orthopedic Institution, known also as the Hospital for the Cure of Deformities of the Human Frame. His contemporary, Dr. Henry Jacob Bigelow, described the capsule of the hip and performed the first reported excision of the hip. This procedure, performed for a patient with severe osteoarthritis, was, in effect, a resection arthroplasty. Dr. Buckminster Brown, son of Dr. John Ball Brown, is thought to be the first American surgeon to devote himself entirely to orthopedics. In 1861 he established the House of the Good Samaritan, which started as an orthopedic institution and many years later was the setting for important contributions to the care and study of rheumatic fever.

Throughout the early decades of the twentieth century, Dr. Robert Lovett had great interest in arthritis. Working in orthopedic surgery at the Children's Hospital, he established what was perhaps the first physical therapy unit in Boston.

Probably, however, Dr. Joel Goldthwait was the first Boston orthopedist to have arthritis as his primary interest. As a staff member at the Massachusetts General Hospital shortly after 1900, he became interested in reconstructive surgery, especially of joints destroyed by tuberculosis. During that period, Dr. Goldthwait spent several years studying and observing at academic centers in northern Italy, where orthopedists had made significant advances in this field. At that time, the notion was widely held in Europe that chronic deforming arthritis might be tubercular in origin. Dr. Goldthwait, however, was concerned with other possible etiologic factors. On his return to Boston in 1909, he began metabolic studies of serum calcium and phosphorous levels in a laboratory in the basement of the Massachusetts General Hospital. Shortly thereafter, he transferred his clinical and research activities to the Carney Hospital in Dorchester, where in 1911 he established one of the earliest arthritis clinics in this country.

While in Cambridge, England with the American expeditionary forces during World War I, he visited the hospital started just before the war by T. S. P. Strangeways. This unique institution combined clinical care of arthritis patients with laboratory research on rheumatic diseases, and Dr. Goldthwait was much impressed with the concept. On returning from military service, Dr. Goldthwait saw the opportunity to have the Robert Breck Brigham Hospital for Incurables develop along the pattern that had so impressed him at the Strangeways, and in this he was successful. In its early years, the emphasis was chiefly orthopedic, with a staff including such outstanding men as Dr. Philip Wilson, Sr., who subsequently headed The Hospital for Special Surgery in New York, Drs. John Kuhns, Loring Swaim, and, later, Theodore Potter and Clement B. Sledge. Dr. Loring Swaim was another orthopedist with primary interest in arthritis. He continued at the Robert Breck Brigham Hospital from 1916 to 1944, was the first Secretary of the American Rheumatism Association, and served as its President in 1941–42.

In spite of the emphasis on orthopedic surgery at the Robert Breck Brigham Hospital, an internist, Dr. Louis Spear, had been appointed as physician-in-chief in 1912, and the role of the nonsurgical staff members was important early in the hospital's development. In those days almost all physicians concerned with the care of rheumatologic patients were internists with a special interest in arthritis. Among these was Dr. Francis C. Hall, who joined the staff in 1925. In the 1920s when the hospital launched its teaching connections with the Harvard Medical School, Boston School of Physical Education, and Boston School of Occupational Therapy, it began to conceive of itself as a research and teaching center and not merely as a home for the so-called incurables. In the 1930s Drs. Spear and Granville A. Bennett, a pathologist whose chief studies were in rheumatic diseases, fostered that point of view. Also at that time, Dr. Marshall Goldthwait Hall, nephew of Dr. Joel Goldthwait, introduced many other young Boston physicians to the staff. Dr. J. Sidney Stillman became chief of the medical service in 1938, and the following year saw the appointments of Drs. Theodore Feldman and Theodore Bayles to the staff. On the staff at the time was Dr. Archibald Nissen, who was particularly interested in the natural history of arthritis. Subsequently, in 1955, Dr. Arthur P. Hall, son of Francis C. Hall, joined the staff as did many others. Dr. Stillman served as President of the ARA in 1971–72.

The excellent programs of research and training begun by these dedicated rheumatologists in the 1930s flourished in the years that followed, particularly after 1966, when Dr. K. Frank Austen was appointed physician-in-chief. In 1980 the long affiliation with the Harvard Medical School was made even stronger with the move of the Robert Breck Brigham Hospital to the Harvard complex of hospitals as a division of the Affiliated Hospital Center.

Beginning in 1932 at the Thorndike Memorial Laboratory of Boston City Hospital, Dr. Chester S. Keefer, on the medical service of Dr. George B. Minot, carried out excellent anatomic studies of joints of normal subjects and those with various forms of arthritis. He also performed biochemical, histologic, and serologic studies of synovial fluid. His reports on gonococcal and other types of pyogenic arthritis were classic examples of clinical research.

Tucson, Arizona. Another city where early interest in arthritis flourished was Tucson, because its warm, dry climate attracted people with chronic illnesses. In 1924 Dr. Bernard Wyatt established in Tucson the Desert Sanitorium, a group of small buildings for the care of patients with tuberculosis and with arthritis. He left a few years later to start the Wyatt Clinic and Research Laboratories, where he was joined by Dr. Robert Hicks and in 1935 by Dr. Harry E. Thompson. In 1926 Dr. Paul Holbrook came to the Desert Sanitorium at the invitation of Dr. Roland Davidson, who had succeeded Dr. Wyatt. Dr. Holbrook was joined by Dr. Donald F. Hill in 1931 and was medical director at the sanitorium until he and Dr. Hill established their own group. Dr. Holbrook was President of ARA during the war years from 1942–46. His important role in the establishment of the Arthritis Foundation is discussed in Chapter 4. Dr. Hill served as President of ARA in 1966–67.

Hot Springs, Arkansas. At the turn of the century, Hot Springs, Arkansas received numerous patients who came to take the cure at the famous springs. Many of these patients were recent Jewish immigrants with very meager funds who turned to the local rabbi for assistance. Attempting to raise the money needed for food, housing, and treatment by local contributions became a serious problem, and the rabbi appealed to B'nai B'rith for help. As a result, the Hot Springs Disbursement Committee was formed to assist these indigent people. As the influx continued, it became apparent that some sort of treatment facility was needed, and after much planning and fundraising, the Leo N. Levi Memorial Hospital opened on November 1, 1914. The initial 20 beds later increased to 112. In 1919 a free outpatient clinic was opened. Although the hospital served as a general one, it developed a particular concern for arthritis and other rheumatic ills because of the large number of patients with arthritis who came to Hot Springs. In 1951, after the establishment of the county hospital and the enlargement of the local Catholic hospital, the Levi Memorial dropped the general hospital role entirely and specialized solely in rheumatic diseases.

Buffalo, New York. In 1929 during his housestaff experience at the Buffalo General Hospital, Dr. L. Maxwell Lockie became interested in arthritis because of the plight of his rheumatologic patients. In the interim between that experience and the start of an assistant residency in medicine at the Johns Hopkins Hospital in 1931, Dr. Lockie visited the few arthritis clinics then in existence in Boston and New York and received encouragement from such men as Drs. Walter Bauer, Ralph Boots, and Russell Cecil, which confirmed his decision to specialize in arthritis. During his year at the Johns Hopkins Hospital, he started an arthritis clinic. On his return to Buffalo in 1932, Dr. Lockie became one of the early physicians in this country to limit his practice to rheumatology. He at once organized an arthritis clinic at the E. J. Meyer Hospital and contributed to teaching at the University of Buffalo School of Medicine. His enthusiasm and dedication made a great impression on colleagues and the public alike, and his role in stimulating interest in rheumatology, not only in western New York, but nationally, was important. He was a founding member of the ARA and served as its President in 1957–58.

Dr. John Talbott entered the Buffalo scene somewhat later when he was appointed Chairman of the Department of Medicine at the University of Buffalo School of Medicine at the end of World War II, but his rheumatologic interests began earlier at the Massachusetts General Hospital. In his junior year at Harvard Medical School, he had begun working in the fatigue laboratory of the Harvard Business School and in the metabolic laboratory of Dr. Arlie V. Bock. After housestaff training at the Presbyterian Hospital in New York City, he returned to work in the two laboratories at Harvard. He became interested in gout as a metabolic problem and, while in Boston, limited his rheumatologic research to that disease. After his move to Buffalo, he expanded his interests to include all types of rheumatic diseases. In later years he became equally well known as a writer of excellent monographs on gout and connective tissue diseases and editor of medical journals including the *Journal of the American Medical Association* and later, *Seminars in Arthritis and Rheumatism.*

Pittsburgh. The pioneer in Pittsburgh was Dr. H. M. Margolis. Like most medical students in the mid-1920s, he had found arthritis a less than appealing subject in his undergraduate days because the views of his teachers on treatment and prognosis were depressing. However, after his experience at the Mayo Clinic as a fellow under Dr. Philip Hench in 1927, his career in rheumatology was established. In 1930 he returned to

Pittsburgh and the practice of internal medicine with primary interest in rheumatology, and by 1936 he was given the opportunity to start an arthritis clinic at the University of Pittsburgh Medical School. This clinic was the forerunner of the outstanding rheumatology unit developed in later years by Dr. Gerald P. Rodnan.

Cleveland. One of the most distinguished figures of the period was Dr. Robert M. Stecher of Cleveland, quoted earlier in this chapter. He was attracted to rheumatology by the severe rheumatoid arthritis of his mother, who made yearly visits to Tucson for treatment. Stecher worked with Holbrook in Tucson for a time and returned to practice rheumatology in Cleveland in 1930. He started an arthritis clinic at Cleveland City Hospital in 1935. He was for years the outstanding figure in Cleveland, where his efforts had laid the foundation for the important program subsequently developed at the Case Western Reserve Medical School by Drs. Paul Vignos and Roland W. Moskowitz. He was long a leader in the affairs of the ARA and was its President in 1947–48. Dr. Stecher was the second American President of the International League Against Rheumatism.

Detroit. Dr. Frank J. Sladen, who had completed his training under Dr. William Osler of Johns Hopkins Hospital, came to Detroit in 1914 on the invitation of Mr. Henry Ford to recruit the staff of the Henry Ford Hospital. Dr. Sladen began a consulting service for patients with arthritis in 1918. In 1925 he was joined by Dr. Dwight C. Ensign who established the Division of Arthritis in 1948. In that year Dr. John W. Sigler joined the staff. Shortly thereafter, one- to two-year fellowships in rheumatology were begun. Dr. Ensign served as division head until 1967 and Dr. Sigler from 1967 to 1982, when he was succeeded by Dr. Howard Duncan.

Chicago. In Chicago the views of Dr. Frank Billings were widely held after his report on focal infection in 1912 (13). After his death, his efforts were carried on by his pupils, Drs. Joseph Miller, Wilbur Post, and Willard Wood. Certainly one of the leaders in medicine in the Chicago area in the 1920s was Dr. Ernest E. Irons, head of the Department of Medicine at Rush Medical College, who, though an internist and not primarily interested in arthritis, was active in the efforts to start an organized campaign against rheumatic diseases. In 1934–35 he served as the first President of the American Association for the Study and Control of Rheumatic Diseases, the forerunner of the ARA. Dr. Evan M. Barton, an intern on his service at the Presbyterian Hospital in Chicago in 1929, was encouraged by Dr. Irons to have additional training abroad. Returning to Chicago in 1935, he was assigned by Dr. Irons to the arthritis clinic.

In the arthritis clinic at Research and Educational Hospital of the University of Illinois, Drs. I. Dreyer and C. I. Reed were engaged in a clinical trial of massive doses of vitamin D for rheumatoid arthritis (37), but this treatment proved ineffective and dangerous and was abandoned after a few years of rather widespread use. In 1933 that clinic was reorganized by Dr. Irving E. Steck. Others active in rheumatology in the 1930s were Drs. David Markson at Northwestern Medical School, George Stuppy at the University of Chicago Clinics, Eugene F. Trout at Cook County Hospital, Emil Vrtiak at the Central Free Dispensary of Rush Medical School, and Drs. Paul S. Carlan and Isidore Pilot.

The 1940s witnessed the arrivals of Drs. Max Montgomery in medicine and Granville Bennett in pathology at the University of Illinois and of Dr. Edward Rosenberg, fresh from a fellowship with Dr. Hench, at the Michael Reese Hospital. In 1947 the Chicago Rheumatism Society was established, with Dr. Rosenberg serving as President. The important developments at Northwestern University under Dr. Frank R. Schmid came after the period covered in this chapter.

San Francisco. In San Francisco Dr. William J. Kerr, a distinguished internist and Chairman of the Department of Medicine at the University of California, had no primary interest in rheumatology but was a man of broad medical interests and influence. He assisted in the early development of ARA and became its first President in 1937–38. He encouraged Dr. Stacy Mettier, a hematologist on his staff, to start an arthritis clinic in 1935. Drs. Frances Baker, an orthopedist, and Salvator P. Lucia, another hematologist, also served on the staff. Dr. Hans Waine became interested in arthritis during his internship at the University of California in 1937 because of a basic interest in chronic illnesses and an unusual rheumatoid arthritis patient with severe systemic features. As a result, he spent two years as a fellow with Dr. Walter Bauer at the Massachusetts General Hospital before returning to the University of California to reorganize the arthritis clinic and start a career in teaching and research. Dr. Waine encouraged Drs. Howard J. Weinberger and Ephraim Engleman to obtain fellowships with Dr. Bauer before he rejoined Bauer's group in Boston in 1949. Dr. Waine also contributed importantly in the development of the Massachusetts Chapter of the Arthritis Foundation. Dr. Weinberger returned to California to practice rheumatology in Los Angeles, and Dr. Engleman replaced Dr. Waine at the University of California in San Francisco. Dr. Engleman was President of the ARA in 1962–63 and President of the International League against Rheumatism in 1981–85. His important roles in the affairs of the ARA, Arthritis Foundation, and NIADDK are discussed in subsequent chapters.

Southern California. In the Los Angeles area, the first internist with a major interest in arthritis appears to have been Dr. David G. Ghrist who came to the Los Angeles General Hospital as an intern in 1925. A fellowship at the Mayo Foundation from 1927 to 1930 included rheumatologic experience under Dr. Philip Hench, with whom he wrote a paper on the course and prognosis in chronic infectious arthritis. He returned to Los Angeles in 1930 to practice internal medicine with major emphasis on rheumatology, as illustrated by his membership in the Society for the Study and Control of Rheumatic Diseases and his contributions to the 1935 *Rheumatism Review.*

Dr. Edward W. Boland also had his first rheumatology training under Dr. Hench at the Mayo Foundation and started practice as an internist with rheumatologic interest in Los Angeles in 1938. During World War II he served with Dr. Hench in establishing the Arthritis Center at the Army and Navy General Hospital at Hot Springs, Arkansas. In the years that followed, he became an indefatigable worker for the American Rheumatism Association and was President in 1954–55. Dr. Carlos Sacasa was a third southern California rheumatologist who received his training at the Mayo Foundation with Drs. Hench and Slocumb. In 1946 he began practice in Pasadena, where among his other rheumatologic services he succeeded, with Dr. Boland, Dr. Nathan Headley, and others, in launching the Southern California Rheumatism Society and the corresponding chapter of the Arthritis Foundation.

Rochester, New York. Dr. William W. Reed, who was in practice in Rochester, New York in the 1830s and 1860s, although not primarily interested in arthritis, made careful anatomic and physiologic studies of the hip joint and its controlling muscles and contributed importantly to the treatment of dislocation of that joint (8). Dr. C. LeRoy Steinberg of that city, about 1930, was one of the first to write on the relationship between ulcerative colitis and ankylosing spondylitis. Other excellent rheumatologists on the staff of the Strong Memorial Hospital were Drs. Stafford Warren and Ralph F. Jacox in the 1940s and subsequently, Dr. John H. Vaughan who was ARA President in 1970–71.

In addition to the early rheumatologists mentioned in these brief summaries, others included Drs. James Craig Small of Philadelphia, Macnider Wetherby of Minneapolis, John W. Gray of Newark, New Jersey, O. O. Ashworth of Richmond, Virginia, and Edward K. Cravener and Millard Smith of Boston. These physicians spoke, along with others previously cited, on the first scientific program of the American Committee for the Control of Rheumatism held in New Orleans on May 9, 1932. It is noteworthy that only the last four papers were on subjects other than foci of infection and the use of vaccines, again illustrating how those subjects dominated rheumatologic thinking in those days.

In this listing of physicians with early concern for arthritis, one may also mention those distinguished men who, though not primarily interested in rheumatic diseases, gave their time and serious thought, as members of the American Committee for the Study and Control of Rheumatism, to the development of an organized effort to combat arthritis. Dr. Ernest Irons has been mentioned as a leader in Chicago. Other physicians were Drs. Russell Haden of Cleveland, Charles Bass of New Orleans, Lewellys Barker of Baltimore, Joseph Miller of Chicago, Rea Smith of Los Angeles, and Ralph Pemberton of Philadelphia as chairman. There were also three orthopedists: Drs. Melvin Henderson of Rochester, Minnesota, Archer O'Reilly of St. Louis, and Robert Osgood of Boston. Subsequently, five members were added: Drs. A. Almon Fletcher of Toronto, Philip Hench of Rochester, Minnesota, and George R. Minot, Cyrus C. Sturgis, and Hans Zinsser of Boston. Of these men, only Drs. Pemberton, Hench, and perhaps Fletcher could be considered true rheumatologists; yet the accomplishments made in this field in the United States since 1928 owe their beginnings to this wise and determined group.

2

The Beginning of the Modern Period

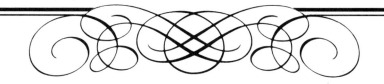

ALTHOUGH all of the physicians and units discussed in Chapter 1 had a significant role in the development of rheumatology during the transition period of the 1920s and 1930s, most significant of all were the contributions made at the Mayo Clinic, Harvard University, Columbia University, New York University, the University of Michigan, and the University of Pennsylvania.

EARLY RHEUMATOLOGIC UNITS

Mayo Clinic. The story at the Mayo Clinic in Rochester, Minnesota starts with Dr. Philip S. Hench. The beginnings have become somewhat legendary. It is said that when Dr. Hench was a resident physician on the service of Dr. Norman Keith, a pioneer in the field of nephrology, they saw a patient at rounds who Dr. Keith thought had degenerative arthritis. Dr. Hench, however, believed that the diagnosis was what was then called chronic infectious arthritis, and he stated his opinion. In those days residents seldom contradicted their supervisors, and Dr. Keith was sufficiently impressed to bring the incident to the attention of Dr. Will Mayo himself. As a result, Dr. Mayo asked Hench if he would like to obtain training in rheumatology and become the Mayo Clinic's expert in that field. Hench accepted eagerly and left for a year of experience in Germany. On his return he was appointed to the staff of the Mayo Clinic on January 1, 1926 with residents assigned to him from the start and, subsequently, fellows.

The importance of that training program, both qualitatively and quantitatively, can scarcely be overstated, for it was at one time the only place in the United States where organized graduate training in rheumatology could be obtained. When Dr. Howard Polley reviewed the 1962–63 membership roster of the ARA, he found that at that time 9.6% of all members had received all or part of their training under Dr. Hench, either at the Mayo

Clinic or during World War II (111). Dr. Hench's roles in the development of the organized effort to combat arthritis and in the discovery of cortisone are discussed in later chapters.

Philip Hench's importance in this training is underscored by the fact that he was the only staff member in rheumatology at the Mayo Clinic until 1935, when he was joined by Dr. Charles Slocumb. Dr. Howard Polley came to the Mayo Clinic in 1942 and Dr. Emmerson Ward in 1950. All three associates of Dr. Hench made important contributions in clinical research and in the affairs of the ARA, serving as Presidents in 1951–52, 1964–65, and 1969–70, respectively.

Although clinical research was actively pursued from the start in 1926 and some of the fellows working for masters degrees carried out laboratory and other studies, in the opinion of Dr. Polley, rheumatologic laboratory research in the modern full-time sense began in 1965 with the appointment of Dr. Frederic McDuffie.

Harvard. The first full-time, university-oriented rheumatology units were the four established at Harvard, Columbia, New York University, and the University of Michigan. The unit at Harvard began in 1929 with the support of a fund established as a memorial to Dr. Robert W. Lovett. As mentioned earlier, Dr. Lovett was a member of the Orthopedic Department at the Harvard Medical School. After his death in 1925, a number of his colleagues and friends, led by Dr. Frank R. Ober, started a fund in his memory, the Robert W. Lovett Memorial for the Study of Crippling Diseases. Although Dr. Lovett's major interest had been in crippling caused by poliomyelitis, the committee in charge selected arthritis as the first field of study in 1929. Dr. Walter Bauer, who was then conducting research on lead poisoning with Dr. Joseph Aub, was recruited to direct the new program. He was at first reluctant to enter such an unpromising field, but in the course of a long and, as he liked to say, somewhat bibulous evening, was persuaded to do so by Dr. Cecil Drinker.

From the start, the unit was concerned equally with care of patients, training, and clinical and laboratory research. The first paper, on normal synovial fluid of cattle, was published in 1930. The Lovett Fund provided salaries, supplies, and some equipment, and the Massachusetts General Hospital gave office and laboratory space as well as clinical facilities. In the first seven years, research grants were made by the Rockefeller and Markle Foundations, and in 1938 a large grant from the Commonwealth Fund became available. With this support, a far-ranging and important research program was undertaken, and it grew in excellence as the years passed.

The training program was equally important. Dr. Charles L. Short joined the unit in 1930 and Dr. Marian W. Ropes in 1932. Drs. Granville A. Bennett and Frederick W. Rhinelander, II, of the Department of Pathology and Drs. Alexander Marble, A. O. Ludwig, Charles F. Warren, and Howard C. Coggeshall of the Department of Medicine were the others in that stimulating group. Most served initially as the equivalent of today's fellows. Over the years, there were hundreds of fellows, many of whom became leaders in rheumatology throughout the world. Dr. Stephen M. Krane became director of this outstanding unit after Dr. Bauer's death in 1963.

Columbia University. The second of the academically oriented rheumatology units was at Columbia University's College of Physicians and Surgeons. The Edward Daniels Faulkner Clinic for Arthritis was established at the Presbyterian Hospital in New York through a fund given by Mrs. Faulkner, with the encouragement of Dr. Fordyce B. St. John, as a memorial to her husband, who had been severely crippled by rheumatoid arthritis. In the spring of 1928, Dr. St. John and Dr. Walter Palmer, Chairman of the Department of Medicine at Columbia, asked Dr. Ralph H. Boots to organize such a clinic. Dr. Boots had done research on rheumatic fever under the direction of Dr. Homer F. Swift at the Rockefeller Institute for Medical Research in New York and later had a medical practice with strong rheumatologic orientation. When the clinic opened in 1929, the initial, part-time staff consisted of Dr. Dumont Elmendorf, clinician; Dr. Robert Muller, specialist in physical medicine; Dr. Mather Cleveland, orthopedic consultant; and Dr. Boots, director. Dr. Martin Henry Dawson joined this group within a few months, serving on a full-time basis. Dr. Dawson, who was recruited from the Rockefeller Institute where he had done microbiologic research on pneumonia with Drs. Oswald Avery and Rufus Cole, immediately started excellent clinical and laboratory research as well as a most productive fellowship program. This unit subsequently made important immunochemical contributions through the research of Michael Heidelberger, PhD and in collaboration with Dr. Harry Rose, Chairman of the Department of Microbiology, leading to recognition of rheumatoid factors.

In 1945 after the death of Dr. Dawson, his place was taken by Dr. Charles Ragan, a staff member who was a former fellow. Dr. Charles Christian, also a former fellow, succeeded Dr. Ragan. After Dr. Christian moved to The Hospital for Special Surgery, his successor was Dr. E. Carwile LeRoy and subsequently Dr. Leonard Chess.

New York University. The third of the four academically oriented units was at New York University. Dr. Currier McEwen, who had his undergraduate and housestaff experience there and at Bellevue Hospital, had, like Dr. Boots, spent four years in research on rheumatic fever with Dr. Homer Swift at the Rockefeller Institute. On his return to New York University in 1932, he immediately started a rheumatologic unit, subsequently called the Rheumatic Diseases Study Group, devoted to patient care, teaching, and clinical and laboratory research in rheumatic fever as well as other rheumatic diseases. This group prospered through the full support of Dr. John H. Wyckoff, Dean and Chairman of the Department of Medicine. A distinctive feature was the unit's organization from the start as an interdepartmental group, with initial members from the departments of medicine, pediatrics, and microbiology and, subsequently, participation by 12 basic science and clinical departments. It differed from other units in that it came about not as the result of stimulus from funds provided by memorial endowments, but from the determined effort of the parent medical school department. Crucial to the success of the Study Group were the encouragement and budgetary support given by Dr. Wyckoff and Dr. McEwen's personal interest because his father, also a physician, had been severely crippled by psoriatic arthritis.

Financial support came almost solely from the departmental budget until the end of World War II, when a sorely needed grant was provided by the Ralph B. Rogers Foundation in 1949. A few years later, support was given by the Masonic Foundation for Medical Research, which began providing similar grants for rheumatologic research to all medical schools in the state of New York.

In 1956 the Masonic Foundation decided to devote all its funds to research on aging. At that critical period, funding for the program at New York University was continued and expanded by one of the first large training grants provided by the then National Institute of Arthritis and Metabolic Diseases (NIAMD). This Institute played a vital role 5 years later in creating new rheumatology units in medical schools throughout the nation through its program-project grants program (see Chapter 10).

In 1933, only a year after the start of the Rheumatic Diseases Study Group, Dr. Joseph J. Bunim joined the staff and continued as a key member of the group for 21 years. He contributed greatly to the excellence of the programs in patient care, teaching, and research until he left in 1954 to become the first Clinical Director and Chief, Arthritis and

Rheumatism Branch of the NIAMD's intramural program in Bethesda, Maryland. Meanwhile, Dr. Morris Ziff had joined in 1950 and stepped into Dr. Bunim's role as scientific catalyst of the team. On Dr. Ziff's departure to head the rheumatology unit at University of Texas, Southwestern Medical School in Dallas in 1958, he was succeeded by Dr. Edward C. Franklin, a former student who had received excellent research experience with Dr. Henry Kunkel at the Rockefeller University. When Dr. McEwen retired as chairman of the group in 1968, Dr. Franklin took over that post. After Dr. Franklin's untimely death in 1982, Dr. Gerald Weissmann was appointed chairman. Others who joined the group on a full-time basis at its first expansion at the end of World War II included Drs. Leon Sokoloff in pathology, Maxwell Schubert in biochemistry of connective tissues, and Alan Bernheimer in microbiology.

Over the years, the fellowship program provided training in laboratory and clinical aspects of rheumatic diseases for more than 200 fellows, many of whom went on to important academic positions in the United States and abroad. Many medical students also took long-term rheumatology electives with the unit. Dr. Elvira DeLill Burke was the first of these in 1935, and she, like others later, went on to a fellowship.

University of Michigan. The fourth of these pioneer academic rheumatology units was at the University of Michigan in Ann Arbor, established in 1937 as the Rackham Arthritis Research Unit. Mrs. Bryson D. Horton, sister of Horace H. Rackham, who had rheumatoid arthritis, was cared for by Dr. Carl Badgly, Chief of the Section of Orthopedic Surgery. Dr. Badgly encouraged her husband, B. D. Horton, executor for the Rackham estate, to establish an endowment for research on arthritis. Dr. Richard Freyberg, who was then involved in research on calcium and phosphorus metabolism with Dr. L. H. Newburgh in the Department of Medicine, was selected to direct the new unit because such studies were considered relevant to arthritis. Dr. Charley J. Smyth joined Dr. Freyberg as his first physician associate in 1938. Dr. Smyth's interest in clinical investigation, teaching, and care of rheumatic patients was continued as Chief of Medicine at Wayne County General Hospital from 1941 to 1949 and then at the University of Colorado in Denver, where he developed and led the important rheumatology program. Dr. Freyberg served as director until 1944, when he became Physician-in-Chief at The Hospital for Special Surgery in New York, and was succeeded by Dr. William D. Robinson. Dr. Ivan F. Duff followed as director at Michigan in 1953 and Dr. Giles G. Bole in 1969. The excellent research and fellowship training at the Rackham Unit contributed much to the infant specialty of rheumatology.

University of Pennsylvania. Although some years later and not developed on an academically full-time basis, the program at the University of Pennsylvania also belongs in this group of pioneer units. Dr. Ralph Pemberton started the first teaching in arthritis for the Graduate School of Medicine at the University of Pennsylvania in the late 1920s and stimulated a number of men to become interested in rheumatology, including Dr. Clyde Kelchner of Allentown and Dr. Morris Bowie of Philadelphia. In 1937 Dr. Bernard I. Comroe started the first arthritis clinic at the Hospital of the University of Pennsylvania, where he also gave lectures on rheumatic diseases to medical students. His most important contribution, however, was the writing of the first accurate, comprehensive textbook on arthritis, *Arthritis and Allied Conditions*. This book, first published in 1940, was an immediate success. A second edition followed in 1942 and a third in 1944.

After the untimely death of Dr. Comroe in 1945, Dr. Perry Pepper, Chairman of the Department of Medicine, persuaded Dr. Joseph Hollander to continue the editorship. Dr. Hollander had become interested in arthritis through the stimulation of Dr. Comroe and Dr.

Jesse Nicholson, head of the orthopedic service at Children's Hospital in Philadelphia. As a result, he started an arthritis clinic at Pennsylvania Hospital in 1937. On the basis of that experience, he was appointed in World War II to the Army Arthritis Center at Ashburn General Hospital and, subsequently, to the Army and Navy Arthritis Center at Hot Springs, Arkansas, where he served under Drs. Philip Hench and Walter Bauer. From this experience, he became fully dedicated to a career in rheumatology. After the war, he returned to the University of Pennsylvania in 1946. With the help of Dr. George Morris Piersol, Chairman of the Department of Physical Medicine, Dr. Hollander obtained some funds and research space to begin a comprehensive unit at the University of Pennsylvania that would combine teaching and research with clinical care. A fellowship program was instituted in 1949, with Dr. Ernest Brown as the first fellow followed by Drs. Ralph Jessar, Charles Brown from Canada, Daniel McCarty, and many others.

The importance of these academically oriented rheumatology units can scarcely be overstated, not only because of their research contributions but also because of their training programs and the improved image they gradually brought to the specialty of rheumatology. The program at the Mayo Clinic had provided many fine practicing rheumatologists; those at the five university units did so too but also trained young physicians for academic careers. To be sure, full-time academic openings were few for these new specialists until some 25 years later, when the large program-project grants from the National Institute of Arthritis and Metabolic Diseases created rheumatology units at medical schools throughout the nation. Nevertheless, a start had been made, and in the intervening years, some of these new rheumatologists found full-time positions, and many added strength to departments of medicine through part-time appointments. The very presence of these young rheumatologists helped enhance the academic acceptance of the specialty. Still more important in this respect was the influence of these units in bringing about more critical criteria for diagnosis and more rational therapy. Even at the Mayo Clinic, the use of vaccines and removal of foci of infection had been continued, but these modes of therapy were not the practice at any of the university units except for some controlled trials, and those useless and indeed harmful forms of treatment gradually lost favor.

THE WAR YEARS

Dr. Ralph Pemberton's interest in rheumatology was stimulated during World War I by his experience caring for soldiers with arthritis. He had been assigned to United States General Hospital Number 9 at Lakewood, New Jersey. Although no military arthritis centers were designated during that war, General Hospital Number 9 functioned as one. Dr. Pemberton had the opportunity to study some 400 soldiers with arthritis and reported his clinical and laboratory observations in a series of papers (107–109). Among the 4,128,479 soldiers in the American Army between April 1, 1917 and December 31, 1919 were records of 92,633 with arthritis, including 33,613 instances of rheumatoid and osteoarthritis, 24,770 of rheumatic fever, 14,764 of nonarticular rheumatism, 7,895 of gonorrheal arthritis, 188 of tuberculous arthritis, and 82 of gout (61). The diagnostic uncertainty of the time is shown by the fact that rheumatoid and osteoarthritis were combined as a single category for statistical purposes.

In view of the large number of rheumatologic cases from 1917 to 1919, special planning was made for the creation of arthritis centers at the start of World War II. Dr. Philip Hench, who joined the army medical corps early in 1942, had several consultations with the

Surgeon General, as did Drs. Walter Bauer and Paul Holbrook, who were also in military service. As a result, plans were made for the establishment of rheumatism centers. Initially, a rheumatic diseases unit was established under Dr. Hench at Camp Carson in Colorado Springs in 1942. That site had been selected because of the high frequency of rheumatic fever among recruits in Colorado. Dr. Howard C. Coggeshall was in charge of the rheumatic diseases division under Dr. Hench. The staff also included Drs. Carlos Sacasa, Darrell Crain, and others. This unit was especially concerned with rheumatic fever, with as many as 200 patients under Dr. Coggeshall's care at one time (26).

Subsequently, a rheumatism center was established at Army and Navy General Hospital, Hot Springs, Arkansas in the fall of 1942, with Dr. Hench as Director of the center and Chief of Medical Services and Dr. Edward W. Boland as Chief of the Section on Rheumatic Diseases. The excellent staff also included Drs. Coggeshall, who had come with Dr. Hench from Camp Carson, Edward Rosenberg, J. O. Finney, Nathan Headley, Richard Smith, and others. The center, which occupied more than half of the 1,725 beds of the hospital, admitted 5,315 rheumatologic patients during the 18 months between January 1944 and June 1946 (61).

Later, as the number of patients exceeded the capacity of the center in Hot Springs, a second rheumatism center was established in McKinney, Texas at the Ashburn General Hospital, affectionately called "aspirin general" by the staff. Dr. John Harvey, an internist from Lexington, Kentucky, was in charge with Dr. David Kydd of Albany, New York as chief of rheumatology and a rheumatologic staff that included Drs. Nathan Abrams, Victor Balboni, Charles Fogarty, Joseph Hollander, Lewis Kolodny, Max Montgomery, Bernard Rogoff, and Wallace Zeller (70).

Although several of these physicians began their military assignments with an established interest in rheumatology, others were stimulated by their experience at the center. Among these was Dr. J. O. Finney, who returned to his home to start the first arthritis clinic at the University of Alabama in Birmingham, which was the forerunner of the excellent unit later led by Drs. Howard L. Holley and J. Claude Bennett.

In addition to these centers designed chiefly for patients with chronic forms of arthritis, others were established for patients with rheumatic fever. These centers were at Birmingham General Hospital, Van Nuys, California; Foster General Hospital, Jackson, Mississippi; and Torney General Hospital, Palm Springs, California. Because the young soldiers had not had much previous exposure to hemolytic streptococcal infections and were suddenly in close contact in the barracks, the attack rate of rheumatic fever was high. In 1942, 1943, and 1944, the numbers of cases recorded by the Army surgeon general's office were about 1,300, 7,000, and 6,000 respectively. Drs. Hugh Morgan, Chester Keefer, Lowell Rantz, and H. O. Robertson guided the programs at these army hospitals, which made significant contributions in the care of patients and in research.

Of particular importance to research on rheumatic fever was the program established at Warren Air Force Base at Cheyenne, Wyoming. Early in the war, an Armed Forces Epidemiologic Board was appointed, whose guiding spirit was Dr. Colin M. Macleod, Chairman of the Department of Microbiology at New York University School of Medicine. Under the aegis of the Board, a streptococcal research laboratory was established at Warren Air Force Base Hospital under the direction of Dr. Charles H. Rammelkamp, Jr. Drs. Floyd W. Denny, Chandler A. Stetson, Jr., Lewis Wannamaker, and others also served there in the care of patients and in laboratory and clinical research. Their work contributed significant information important to the understanding and management of hemolytic streptococcal infections and rheumatic fever.

The war preempted the best efforts of all citizens, and most rheumatologists throughout the country were in military service or otherwise involved in the war effort. Fuller discussion of the rheumatologic aspects of military medical experience during World War II are given in the publication of the US Army Center of Military History, edited by Dr. W. Paul Havens, Jr. (59).

3

Beginning of the Campaign Against Rheumatism and the Formation of the American Rheumatism Association

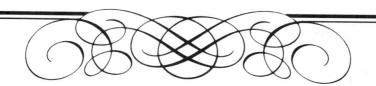

To conduct a successful campaign against a public health problem is an enormous task that requires the organized effort of many dedicated persons. Stimulus to start such a campaign, however, is usually provided by a single physician who recognizes the need and pursues the task with undaunted confidence in success. Such is the case with the campaign against arthritis and rheumatism, the origin of which is generally credited to Dr. Jan van Breemen, a Dutch physician active in the study and treatment of chronic rheumatism in the first decades of the twentieth century (Figure 3-1). Accounts of the early efforts primarily come directly from van Breemen because the written records were destroyed in the invasion of the Netherlands during World War II.

Van Breemen relates (159) that the European campaign against rheumatism was conceived during the First International Congress on Physical Treatment held in Berlin in 1913. At this meeting van Breemen presented a report, "French and German Rheumatism and Its Treatment." During discussions in the Congress, van Breemen proposed that a worldwide effort be made to study and control the rheumatic diseases and that an International Institute for Scientific Research of the Rheumatic Diseases be created "to facilitate the obtaining of reports from various countries for the next Congress scheduled to be held in St. Petersburg in 1917." This proposal was adopted but it never materialized; World War I intervened.

At the annual meeting of the International Society of Medical Hydrology held in Paris in 1925, van Breemen's proposal was reexamined, and it was agreed that an International Committee on Rheumatism should be created. To organize this, a committee of physicians was appointed, composed of: Drs. J. Fortescue Fox, London, Chairman; Jan van Breemen, Amsterdam, Secretary; V. Coates, Bath; F. Kormann, Ragaz; and L. Schmidt, Pistany. This committee formulated these objectives:

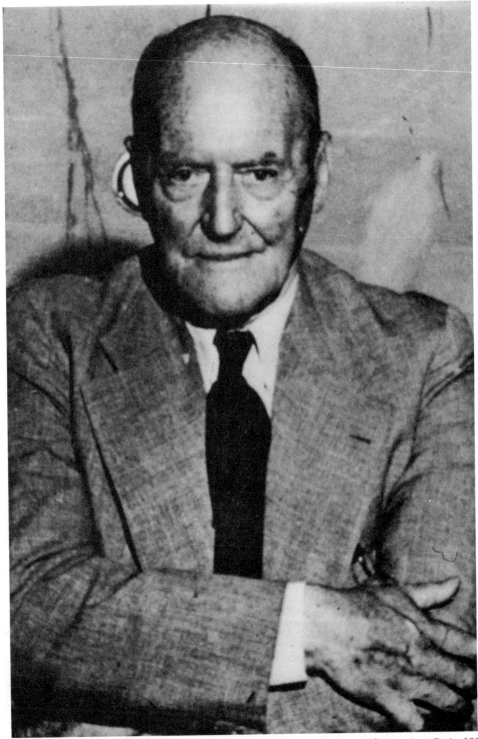

Figure 3-1. Jan van Breemen. Founder of the International League Against Rheumatism. Paris, 1925.

1. That the International Committee on Rheumatism be the central consultative body in an international campaign against rheumatism
2. That the Committee encourage and assist in the formation of national committees against rheumatism
3. That it prepare and circulate statistics on prevalence of various rheumatic diseases, and other pertinent information, in the *Archives of Medical Hydrology* and other appropriate journals

At the next meeting of the International Society of Hydrology, held in Paris in 1927, the report of the organizing committee was received and its recommendations were accepted. The International Committee Against Rheumatism was organized, consisting of Drs. Fox, London, President; J. van Breemen, Amsterdam, Secretary; Jonkheer van Lennep, Amsterdam, Treasurer; and Drs. Dietrich, Berlin; Jacques Forestier, Paris; I. Gunzburg, Antwerp; H. Jansen, Copenhagen; G. Kahlmeter, Stockholm; F. Kormann, Ragaz; L. Schmidt, Pistany; and A. Strasser, Vienna. A central office was established at 489 Keizergracht, Amsterdam. The Committee adopted the motto, "All important social illnesses should be attacked at their source, not fought at their end" (141).

Interest in the rheumatic diseases grew rapidly in Europe. During 1927 and 1928 national committees on rheumatism were formed in Austria, Czechoslovakia, Denmark, France, Great Britain, Germany, Hungary, the Netherlands, Norway, Spain, Sweden, and the U.S.S.R. The Ligue Belge contre le Rhumatisme had been formed in 1926. In 1928 the International Committee Against Rheumatism reorganized under the name of *le Ligue International contre le Rhumatisme* and began conducting its program of activities under the direction of a council composed of: Fox, President; Dietrich, Vice President; van Breemen, Secretary and Director of the Consultative Bureau; Gunzburg, Assistant Secretary. A constitution and bylaws were adopted, and publication of the official journal of the Ligue, *Acta Rheumatologica*, was begun. In an editorial in the first issue of *Acta*, van Breemen stated, "The fight against rheumatic afflictions had to be put on a sound and scientific basis to try to change the ideas prevalent in medical official circles of most countries regarding the importance of these diseases" (106).

BEGINNING OF THE CAMPAIGN AGAINST RHEUMATISM IN THE UNITED STATES

Stimulus for creating a national campaign against rheumatism in the United States came directly from the European International Committee Against Rheumatism. How did the effort in Europe spread to the United States? In the summer of 1926 Dr. Louis B. Wilson, Director of the Mayo Foundation for Medical Education and Research, discussed the problems of rheumatism at length with Drs. Fox and van Breemen while visiting medical centers in Europe. These physicians impressed upon Dr. Wilson the importance of arousing sufficient interest to organize an American committee to join the European committees in the fight against rheumatism, under the aegis of the International Committee Against Rheumatism.

On his return to the United States, Dr. Wilson discussed this proposal with Dr. Philip S. Hench, who was head of the section of rheumatic diseases at the Mayo Clinic. Dr. Hench was enthusiastic and positive. Thereupon, Dr. Wilson corresponded with a small number of American physicians who might, on a priori grounds, be expected to have constructive viewpoints on this matter. This group of doctors included: Drs. Llewellys F. Barker, Baltimore; Charles G. Bass, New Orleans; Russell L. Cecil, New York; Russell L.

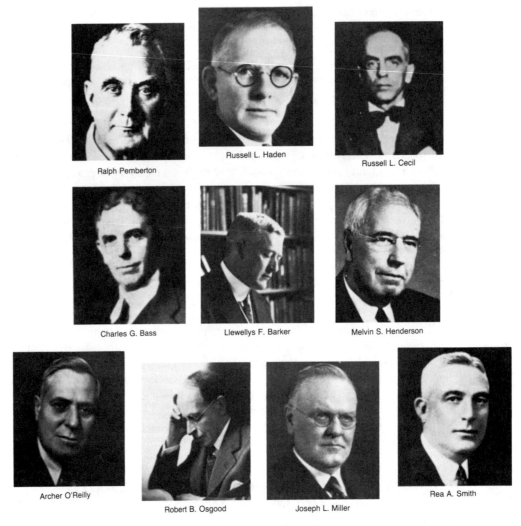

Figure 3-2. Organizing Committee for the American Committee Against Rheumatism.

Haden, Kansas City; Melvin S. Henderson, Rochester, Minnesota; Joseph L. Miller, Chicago; Archer O'Reilly, St. Louis; Robert B. Osgood, Boston; Ralph Pemberton, Philadelphia; and Rea A. Smith, Los Angeles. Dr. Pemberton was asked to serve as chairman of this 10-physician group, which was requested to organize an *American Committee Against Rheumatism* as part of the International League (140) (Figure 3-2).

    These men were not convened as a committee until Dr. Pemberton studied the matter further. He went to Europe in 1927 and spent days with van Breemen discussing progress in the fight against rheumatism and future directions. He then visited England, where he talked at length with Fox, Sir Humphrey Rolleston, and other British physicians active in the field of arthritis. He came away impressed that earnest, knowledgeable, and influential men were engaged in this worthwhile cause. He was eager to pursue the challenge of getting the American Committee organized and active.

After his return from Europe, Dr. Pemberton spent several months corresponding with Dr. Wilson and discussing with the physicians on the original committee how best to proceed. He related that Dr. Osgood, an outstanding Boston orthopedist who had become interested in the crippling resulting from chronic arthritis, was particularly helpful. It was apparent to both Drs. Pemberton and Osgood that the fight against rheumatism belonged in the category of internal medicine, that no other field could constitute the premise from which a broad-gauged approach should be launched.

As chairman, Dr. Pemberton called a meeting of the original committee on March 17, 1928 in Philadelphia. Drs. Bass, Cecil, Haden, Henderson, Miller, O'Reilly, Osgood, and Pemberton attended. This was the first official meeting of American physicians attempting to create a widespread interest in rheumatism and to plan for study and treatment of the rheumatic diseases. The group decided to call itself *The American Committee for the Control of Rheumatism*. The following physicians were added to the Committee: Drs. A. Almon Fletcher, Toronto, Canada; Philip S. Hench, Rochester, Minnesota; George R. Minot, Boston; Cyrus C. Sturgis, Boston; and Hans Zinsser, Boston. Hench later was elected Secretary.

EARLY ACTIVITIES OF THE AMERICAN COMMITTEE FOR THE CONTROL OF RHEUMATISM

Dr. Pemberton was designated to write an editorial for the *Journal of the American Medical Association* to explain why the American Committee for the Control of Rheumatism was established, its purposes, and European progress in the fight against rheumatism. The editorial appeared in the July 7, 1928 issue. Its forcefulness is shown by this quote:

> The magnitude of the problem will not permit an early solution, but plans have been laid for arousing the interest of the medical men as well as the lay public in the importance of the subject. Among matters of primary interest are systematization of nomenclature and other matters fundamental to the interchange of ideas; the compilation of statistics; the development of coordinated research; the evaluation of various forms of treatment; the better education of the medical student in regard to the disease; and the extrusion of information among practitioners regarding the rheumatoid problem and the existing therapeutic measures of proved value (105).

A subcommittee composed of Drs. Osgood, Haden, and Cecil prepared a booklet suitable for physicians and the laity, outlining the prevalence of arthritis, its economic importance, and the comparative neglect endured by patients with chronic arthritis. The booklet was printed and widely distributed by the Metropolitan Life Insurance Company in 1930, under the title "What is Rheumatism?" (164). This same company had published a pamphlet in 1927 titled "Rheumatic Diseases," with a quote on the last page from the famous clinician and medical educator, Dr. Thomas McCrae: "Knowledge of the chronic diseases of the joints is in an unsatisfactory condition, and great differences of opinion exist on many points" (117).

The minutes of early meetings of the American Committee record many discussions concerning plans for promoting research, establishing arthritis clinics, influencing the teaching of rheumatic disease in medical schools, increasing membership of the Committee, hiring an executive secretary, and obtaining funding for the Committee's activities. In

1929 the Committee felt the time had come to enlist economic support from laypersons, and indeed, some money was collected.

During a meeting of the Committee held in Kansas City, October 10, 1929, it was decided to display exhibits, primarily to educate physicians on the diagnosis and differentiation of common forms of arthritis and accepted modalities of treatment. These displays at first were shown in the scientific exhibit section of the annual sessions of the American Medical Association. The first exhibit was at the 1930 Detroit session, the second, in Philadelphia in 1931, the third, in New Orleans in 1932, and the last, in Cleveland in 1934. Many physicians visited these exhibits, which did much to arouse interest in rheumatic diseases.

Other educational exhibits were prepared for the public to emphasize the ravages of rheumatic illnesses and the need for an intensive crusade to combat them. A special exhibit for laypeople was prepared for the "Century of Progress" World's Fair in Chicago, which ran from June to November 1933. Informational literature was distributed to the viewers of the exhibit.

Another early step taken by the Committee was to inform the medical profession and the public regarding basic concepts of chronic arthritis. This they did by preparing and distributing a small card that read:

Concept Of American Committee For The
Control Of Rheumatism Concerning The Disease Commonly
Called Chronic Rheumatism Or Arthritis

1. The disease is chronic, prevalent in all temperate zones and represents one of the most important, if not *the* most important of existing social and industrial handicaps.
2. The Committee conceives of the disease as a generalized illness with joint manifestations. Certain prodromes may be recognized and it is of vital importance that they be recognized.
3. It is the opinion of the Committee that at the present time no single infectious agent or any completely defined dietary deficiency or metabolic disturbance has been conclusively shown to be the sole cause of these disorders. The Committee inclines to the belief that any one of these factors, under appropriate circumstances, may basically underlie the onset of the disease.
4. The Committee feels it is of vital importance that the medical profession have its attention directed to the methods of treatment and proved value which are at present at its disposal. In spite of etiological uncertainties, the Committee feels that properly managed therapy which takes into account both infectious and metabolic factors has yielded results which encourage optimism and impose the obligation of further developing such methods.
5. In the light of the foregoing considerations, the Committee proposes to broadcast, as widely as possible, both to the profession and to the public its concept of the nature of the types of arthritis included under the heading chronic rheumatism, its belief as to the probable predisposing and existing causes of the disease and the knowledge which the Committee possesses or may acquire as to the most efficient methods of treatment.

In a draft of the concept card was a sixth statement, an opinion often expressed by Dr. Pemberton but not generally accepted:

It is the belief of the Committee that optimism rather than pessimism should dominate the attitude of the profession toward this problem. In most cases the treatment would represent a combination of various coordinated measures of therapy rather than a single procedure. Experience leads to the belief that under such circumstances an attitude of optimism toward the control of the problem is justified.

That this statement was controversial was indicated by its omission from the concepts published on the card.

An important early task of the American Committee was the classification and nomenclature of the rheumatic diseases. Members of the Committee held diverse opinions. After numerous discussions, it was agreed that the classification based on anatomic and pathologic differences published by Nichols and Richardson in 1909 (98), would be a starting point and that a subcommittee of Drs. Cecil, Osgood, and Pemberton should define the classification further. The subcommittee recognized that the terms "proliferative" and "degenerative" arthritis as used by Drs. Nichols and Richardson were synonymous with the British terms "rheumatoid" and "osteoarthritis," respectively.

ANNUAL OPEN MEETINGS OF AMERICAN COMMITTEE BEGIN

The first open scientific meeting sponsored by the American Committee was a conference held on May 9, 1932, immediately preceding the annual session of the American Medical Association in New Orleans. Announcement of this meeting in the *Journal of the American Medical Association* (28) read: "A Conference on Rheumatic Diseases, an open meeting sponsored by the American Committee for the Study and Control of Rheumatic Diseases." This conference was the first scientific meeting in America devoted wholly to the subject of rheumatism. Dr. Pemberton was chairman; eleven papers were presented. The titles of these papers reflect much of the thinking concerning the rheumatic diseases 50 years ago (Figure 3-3).

In the chairman's opening address, Dr. Pemberton reviewed the events that led to the formation of the American Committee and stated its purposes. The first scientific paper dealt with the clinical and economic aspects of arthritis. A paper presented by Dr. Hench (coauthored by Dr. Judd, surgeon in the Mayo Clinic) was "Gallbladder Disease in Chronic Infectious Arthritis: Results of Cholecystectomy." Dr. Holbrook (of Tucson) discussed climate as a factor in treatment of chronic arthritis. Note the subject of paper number 6, "Desensitization Treatment (via vaccine) of Chronic Arthritis" and of number 7, "Intravenous Streptococcic Vaccine Therapy."

The missionary role of the Committee is reflected in the "cordial invitation" to visit the display in the scientific exhibit section of the annual session of the American Medical Association. Names of many of the participants in this first conference reappeared often in following years.

The programs for these early conferences were printed several weeks before the conference and sent to departments of medicine, surgery, and physical therapy, to libraries of all medical schools in North America, and to individual physicians and scientists the Committee thought would, or should, be interested in rheumatism.

The second conference sponsored by the American Committee was held in 1933 in Milwaukee. It was, again, a three-hour session and was listed as "an open meeting." As in the first conference, most of the participants in the second conference were leaders in medical education and clinical investigation: Drs. Keefer, Professor of Medicine, Harvard Medical School, later President of the American College of Physicians; R. Ghormley, renowned orthopedic surgeon, Mayo Clinic; Bauer, Professor of Medicine, Harvard Medical School and

PROGRAM

Conference on Rheumatic Diseases

AN OPEN MEETING SPONSORED BY

The American Committee for the Control of Rheumatism

MONDAY, MAY 9, 1932, NINE O'CLOCK A.M. TO TWELVE NOON

Hotel Roosevelt, Room A, New Orleans

It is requested that papers be presented in abstract, not read. Time limit for papers will be 12 minutes. (For total discussion of any one paper time limit 8 minutes). Discussions of any paper by members of the audience are cordially invited.

---

1. Chairman's Introduction—Dr. Ralph Pemberton, Philadelphia

2. "Clinical and Economic Factors of Arthritis in 450 Ex-members of the Military Service.".........
   ....Dr. Philip B. Matz, Washington, D. C.

   Discussion: Dr. Wallace S. Duncan, Cleveland, Ohio, and Dr. Francis C. Hall, Boston.

3. "Relation of the Digestive Tract to Chronic Arthritis"
   ....Dr. T. Preston White, Charlotte, North Carolina

4. "Gallbladder Disease in Chronic Infectious Arthritis: Results of Cholecystectomy".............Dr. E. Starr Judd (and Dr. Philip S. Hench), Rochester, Minnesota

   Discussion (papers No. 3 and No. 4): Dr. R. Garfield Snyder, New York City, and Dr. A. R. Shands, Jr., Durham, North Carolina.

Figure 3-3. Program of first conference on rheumatic diseases in the United States.

an outstanding early investigator of arthritis; Dawson and Boots, Professors of Medicine, College of Physicians and Surgeons, Columbia University; Fletcher, a leading Canadian internist; Key, Professor of Surgery (Orthopedics), Washington University Medical School; Kerr, Professor of Medicine, University of California Medical College; Minot, Professor of Medicine, Harvard Medical School, a Nobel laureate. Without doubt, the successful organization of the American fight against rheumatism, the rapid growth of the movement, and the many accomplishments of the American Committee (later, the American Rheumatism Association) all resulted from the good fortune of having such highly respected leaders in the medical profession collaborating diligently in the campaign during the early years.

The papers presented at the second conference dealt with such diverse subjects as the analgesic effect of hepatitis and jaundice on arthritis and rheumatic pain (Dr. Hench)

5. "Climate Therapy for Chronic Arthritis: Results in 500 Cases"..............Dr. W. Paul Holbrook, Tucson, Arizona

6. "The Desensitization Treatment of Chronic Arthritis"............Dr. James Craig Small, Philadelphia

7. "Intravenous Streptococcic Vaccine Therapy in Chronic Arthritis"............Dr. Macnider Wetherby, Minneapolis

    Discussion (papers No. 5, No. 6 and No. 7) : Dr. John W. Gray, Newark, New Jersey; Dr. Wm. J. Kerr, San Francisco, California, and Dr. O. O. Ashworth, Richmond, Virginia

Papers to be read if time permits

8. "Sinus Infections as Silent Foci in Arthritis"........
................................Dr. R. Garfield Snyder, New York

9. "Degenerative Arthritis in Ilio-femoral Ligaments"........................Dr. Edward K. Cravener, Boston

10. "The Joints in Infection"........Dr. Chester S. Keefer, and Dr. Walter K. Meyers, Boston ....

11. "The Arthritis Problem"........Dr. Millard Smith, Boston

12. "Classification of Osteo-arthritis"..............................
..............................Dr. Walter Gay Lough, New York City

---

You are cordially invited to visit the exhibit of the American Committee for The Control of Rheumatism to be held in Booths 1004, 1006, 1008 and 1010 in the Exhibit Hall.

Ralph Pemberton, M. D., Philadelphia, *Chairman*
Charles C. Bass, M. D., New Orleans
Russell L. Cecil, M. D., New York
A. Almon Fletcher, M. D., Toronto
Russell L. Haden, M. D., Cleveland
Melvin S. Henderson, M. D., Rochester, Minnesota

Joseph L. Miller, M. D., Chicago
George R. Minot, M. D., Boston
J. Archer O'Reilly, M. D., St. Louis
Robert B. Osgood, M. D., Boston
Cyrus C. Sturgis, M. D., Ann Arbor
Hans Zinsser, M. D., Boston
Philip S. Hench, M. D., Rochester, Minnesota, *Secretary*

and trauma as an etiologic factor in arthritis (Dr. Key). New terminology appeared: "degenerative arthritis" and chronic "atrophic (rheumatoid) arthritis." Composition of the American Committee remained the same except for the addition of Dr. Ralph Boots.

AMERICAN RHEUMATISM ASSOCIATION FORMED

In 1933 the American Committee met at least three times. According to the minutes of the meeting held on January 28, members discussed for the first time the formation of an "American Association for the Control of Rheumatism" that would "communicate data on the disease, assist in the raising of funds and support activities designed to prevent and treat the disease." In the June 11 meeting, the Committee drew up plans to organize the association. These early plans provided for membership in the Association to be limited to

Program

Papers will be presented in abstract, not read. Time limit for papers will be 15 minutes. Discussions of any papers by members of the audience are cordially invited.

1. **Arthur Steindler, Iowa City**
   Focal Infection in Arthritis.

2. **Charles W. Wainwright, Baltimore**

   Arthritis and Streptococci Vaccine Based on Skin Sensitivity
   Discussion: (papers 1 and 2) J. Albert Key, St. Louis; M. H. Dawson, New York; Russell L. Cecil, New York; Russell L. Haden, Cleveland.

3. **Frank J. Sladen, Dwight C. Ensign, Clark M. McColl, Detroit**
   Nutritional Factors in Chronic Arthritis.

4. **Frank R. Ober and William T. Green, Boston**
   Arthritis in Children.

5. **W. Paul Holbrook, Tucson**

   Variations in Management during the Different Phases of Atrophic Arthritis.
   Discussion: (papers 3, 4 and 5) Robert B. Osgood, Boston; Ernest E. Irons, Chicago.

6. **C. W. Scull and Ralph Pemberton, Philadelphia**

   The Influence of Dietetic and Other Factors on the Reduction of Swelling of Tissues in Arthritis.
   Discussion: A. Almon Fletcher, Toronto; W. J. Kerr, San Francisco.

7. **Joseph Kovacs, New York**

   The Peripheral Blood Circulation in Chronic Arthritis and the Influence of Vasodilators.
   Discussion: Philip S. Hench, Rochester, Minn.; Irving S. Wright, New York.

8. **John G. Kuhns and H. L. Wetherford, Boston**

   The Role of the Reticulo-Endothelial System in the Deposition of Colloidal Dyes and Particulate Matter in Articular Cavities.
   Discussion: W. J. Kerr, San Francisco; Robert B. Osgood, Boston; Joseph Kovacs, New York.

Figure 3-4. Program of first scientific meeting sponsored by the American Rheumatism Association, 1934.

approximately 100 persons consisting of: 1) physicians who had deep and sincere interest in the study of rheumatic disease and those who had made definite contributions to its literature and 2) physicians and laymen who held positions of influence in public health and medical administration. The American Committee was to act as the "advisory council" to the association. In November 1933, the Advisory Council held its first meeting. The plan for formation of the association was adopted, and some time between this meeting and June 1934, the new Association was formed. The American Committee became the *American Association for the Control of Rheumatism*, according to Stecher (141), but on programs of subsequent annual conferences the name appears as "American Association for the Study and Control of Rheumatic Diseases."

Papers to be read if time permits

9. L. Maxwell Lockie and Roger Hubbard, Buffalo

> Studies on Metabolism of a Case of Gout.
> Discussion: Philip S. Hench, Rochester, Minn.; Francis
> C. Hall, Boston.

10. Edward F. Hartung, New York

> Calcium and Cholesterol Metabolism in Arthritis.
> Discussion: Ralph Pemberton, Philadelphia.

11. G. Douglas Taylor, A. B. Ferguson and Haig Kasabach,
New York

> A Study of Roentgenological Findings in Various Forms
> of Chronic Arthritis.
> Discussion: M. H. Dawson, New York; R. H. Boots, New
> York.

You are cordially invited to the movie exhibit of the American
Committee for the Control of Rheumatism to be held in Booths 532
and 532R at Exhibit Hall.

OFFICERS

ERNEST E. IRONS, M.D., Chicago, *President*

RUSSELL L. HADEN, M.D., Cleveland, *Vice-President*

LORING T. SWAIM, M.D., Boston, *Secretary-Treasurer*

ADVISORY COUNCIL
American Committee for the Control of Rheumatism

RALPH PEMBERTON, M.D., Philadelphia, *Chairman*

PHILIP S. HENCH, M.D., Rochester, Minn., *Secretary*

RALPH H. BOOTS, M.D., New York

A. ALMON FLETCHER, M.D., Toronto

RUSSELL L. CECIL, M.D., New York

RUSSELL L. HADEN, M.D., Cleveland

JOSEPH L. MILLER, M.D., Chicago

GEORGE R. MINOT, M.D., Boston

J. ARCHER O'REILLY, M.D., St. Louis

ROBERT B. OSGOOD, M.D., Boston

CYRUS C. STURGIS, M.D., Ann Arbor

HANS ZINSSER, M.D., Boston

From the time it was organized, the Association took over the work of the American Committee and became the leading force in the American campaign against rheumatism. At its first business meeting, the Association elected these physicians to be its first officers: Drs. Ernest E. Irons, Chicago, President; Russell L. Haden, Cleveland, Vice President; Loring T. Swaim, Boston, Secretary-Treasurer. The members of the American Committee were designated to be the Advisory Council (later the executive committee). The Council agreed to continue the annual scientific conferences in conjunction with the annual sessions of the American Medical Association. Further, it was decided that the Association should prepare a review of literature dealing with arthritis and rheumatism and that this be updated at frequent intervals, annually if possible. Dr. Philip Hench was appointed chairman of the Committee to edit these reviews. This started the most valuable series of reviews of the rheumatism literature published in the English language, the *Rheumatism Reviews*, as the

: Program :

Papers will be presented in abstract, not read. Time limit for papers will be 12 minutes. Discussions of any papers by members of the audience are cordially invited.

Morning Session, nine o'clock

Introductory Remarks
ERNEST E. IRONS, President, Chicago

1. Accelerating Factors in Chronic Degenerative Arthritis
   RUSSELL L. HADEN and W. A. WARREN, Cleveland
   Discussion: WALTER BAUER, Boston

2. Bacteriologic and Serologic Findings in a Group of Patients with Arthritis
   CURRIER McEWEN, New York
   Discussion: RUSSELL L. CECIL, New York

3. Protein Studies in Rheumatoid and Hypertrophic Arthritis
   JOHN STAIGE DAVIS, JR., New York
   Discussion: RALPH PEMBERTON, Philadelphia; RALPH H. BOOTS, N. Y.

4. Further Studies on the Roentgenologic Findings in Various Forms of Chronic Arthritis
   A. B. FERGUSON, HAIG KASABACH and G. DOUGLAS TAYLOR, New York
   Discussion: JOHN G. KUHNS, Boston

5. Home Treatment of Chronic Arthritis by Physiotherapy
   JOHN S. COULTER, Chicago (by invitation)
   Discussion: FRANK R. OBER, Boston

6. Chronic Arthritis; Effect of High Carbohydrate Diet and Insulin on Symptoms and Respiratory Metabolism
   BYRON D. BOWEN and L. MAXWELL LOCKIE, Buffalo
   Discussion: CHARLES W. SCULL, ELKINS PARK, Pa.; T. PRESTON WHITE, Charlotte, N. C.

7. Results of Fever Therapy for Gonorrheal Arthritis, Chronic Infectious (Atrophic) Arthritis, and Other Forms of "Rheumatism"
   PHILIP S. HENCH, Rochester, Minnesota
   Discussion: W. J. STAINSBY, New York; WALTER BAUER, Boston

8. What Can be expected from Orthopaedic Care of Chronic Arthritis
   LORING T. SWAIM, Boston
   Discussion: A. R. SHANDS, JR., Durham, N. C.; DENIS S. O'CONNOR, New Haven

PAPERS TO BE READ IF TIME PERMITS

9. The Treatment of Rheumatoid Arthritis with Leucocyte Cream
   EDWARD F. HARTUNG, New York
   Discussion: M. H. Dawson, New York

Figure 3-5. Program of the second Annual Meeting sponsored by the ARA, Atlantic City, 1935.

series came to be known (see Chapter 7). The Council voted to contribute $100 to *le Ligue International contre le Rhumatisme* to fulfill its obligation to support the international campaign against rheumatism. A corporate seal was adopted.

The third conference on rheumatic diseases was held in Cleveland, June 11, 1934,

10. The Use of Cincophen and its Derivatives in the Treatment of Chronic Arthritis
    R. GARFIELD SNYDER, C. H. TRAEGER, CARL A. ZOLL, LEMOYNE C. KELLY and FRANZ LUST, New York
    Discussion: HOMER F. SWIFT, New York

. . . .

Business Meeting, twelve o'clock

Afternoon Session, two o'clock

1. The Nature of Rheumatic Fever
   HOMER F. SWIFT, New York

2. The Natural History of Childhood Rheumatism in Minnesota
   M. J. SHAPIRO, Minneapolis
   Discussion: (papers 1 and 2) JOHN WYCKOFF, New York, and RALPH KINSELLA, St. Louis

3. The Relationship between Rheumatic Fever and Rheumatoid Arthritis
   M. H. DAWSON and T. L. TYSON, New York
   Discussion: CURRIER MCEWEN, New York, and JOHN R. PAUL, New Haven

4. The Geographical Distribution of Rheumatic Fever and Rheumatic Heart Disease in the United States
   E. STERLING NICHOL, Miami
   Discussion: C. C. MCLEAN, Birmingham, Ala., and T. DUCKETT JONES, Boston

5. Studies Relating to Vitamin C Deficiency in Rheumatic Fever
   JAMES F. RINEHART, San Francisco
   Discussion: HOMER F. SWIFT, New York; M. J. SHAPIRO, Minneapolis, and WILLIAM J. KERR, San Francisco

6. Influence of the Tonsils on Rheumatic Infection in Children
   ALBERT D. KAISER, Rochester, New York
   Discussion: RUSSELL L. CECIL, New York

7. Institutional Provisions for the Care of the Rheumatic Child
   HUGH MCCULLOCH, St. Louis
   Discussion: W. D. STROUD, Philadelphia

8. Fever Therapy in Chorea
   LUCY PORTER SUTTON and KATHERINE DODGE, New York
   Discussion: PHILIP S. HENCH, Rochester, Minnesota; T. DUCKETT JONES, Boston, and JOHN WYCKOFF, New York

this time sponsored by the newly formed American Rheumatism Association. It was listed as the "First Annual Meeting of the American Association for the Study and Control of Rheumatic Diseases." Papers presented dealt with a variety of treatment modalities, etiologic factors, juvenile arthritis, and pathologic physiology in patients with arthritis (Figure 3-4).

The second Annual Meeting of the Association, the fourth conference on rheumatic diseases, took place in Atlantic City in June 1935. This was the first full-day session. A variety of subjects, mostly clinical, made up the morning program. The afternoon session dealt chiefly with rheumatic fever. Again, most of the persons presenting and discussing papers were nationally prominent internists, surgeons, and clinical investigators, all leading figures in the medical profession, including Drs. Boots, Cecil, Dawson, Haden, Hench, Jones, Kerr, Lockie, McEwen, McLean, Nickol, Ober, Paul, Stroud, Swaim, and Swift (Figure 3-5). Two important new names appeared on the Advisory Council—Drs. Walter Bauer and Homer Swift.

In May 1936 the Third Annual Meeting of the Association was held in Kansas City. The program for this Fifth Conference on Rheumatic Disease was unique in that it had an international flavor. Lord Horder, a representative of the British Committee for the Study of Rheumatic Diseases, reviewed "The British Activities for the Control of Rheumatism." The remainder of the program was devoted to diagnosis: one presentation discussed general diagnosis of joint diseases and the remaining 10 papers concerned differential diagnosis of different types of arthritis and nonarticular rheumatism. All were presented by leading academicians. This program may well have been the springboard for the development of the American Rheumatism Association diagnostic criteria. (See Chapter 7.) Indeed, in the following year, Dr. Russell Cecil spoke on "The Necessity of Certain Criteria for the Diagnosis and Cure of Rheumatoid Arthritis" in his presidential address to the American Association for the Study and Control of Rheumatic Diseases.

In 1937 the name of the American Association for the Study and Control of Rheumatic Diseases was changed to *American Rheumatism Association* (ARA) , and it is so listed for the first time on the 1938 annual meeting program.

The scientific programs for the 1938 and 1939 annual Association meetings included a wider variety of topics such as structure and function of synovial membrane and synovial fluid, the physiology and pathology of connective tissue, and evaluation of a range of treatments for arthritis: sulfa drugs, gold preparations, sulfur, vaccines, analgesics, anesthetic injections, physical therapy modalities, and surgical procedures.

In the 1940 scientific session held in New York City, Dr. Philip Hench described palindromic rheumatism in his president's address under the title (so typical of Dr. Hench), "An Oft-Recurring Disease of Joints (Arthritis, Peri-Arthritis, Para-Arthritis) Apparently Producing no Articular Residues: Its Relationship to Angio-neural Arthrosis, Allergic Arthritis and Atrophic Arthritis. Report of Thirty-Four Cases," almost the entire paper presented in the title! The program also listed the arthritis clinics then existing in greater New York; there were 18 in Manhattan and the Bronx and seven in Brooklyn-Queens, an impressive number at this early stage in the American campaign against rheumatism.

RUMBLINGS OF WORLD WAR II SLOW THE CAMPAIGN

In 1940 the American Committee of the International League Against Rheumatism issued a report to American physicians on January 1, titled "Postponed Seventh International Congress on Rheumatic Diseases." The Congress was to have been held in June 1940. This report described elaborate plans for the Congress, with meetings to be held in New York, Philadelphia, and Boston, and explained that "because of the present uncertainty of political relationships among the European nations, it would be unwise to attempt, and probably impossible to hold, a successful Congress in the United States in 1940. Regretfully, therefore, it seems best to postpone this meeting until the European horizon widens." The

American Association for the Study and Control of Rheumatic Diseases

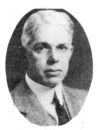
Ernest F. Irons
1934–35

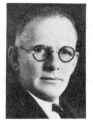
Russell L. Haden
1935–36

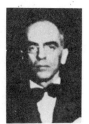
Russell L. Cecil
1936–37

American Rheumatism Association

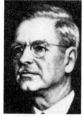
William J. Kerr
1937–38

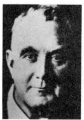
Ralph Pemberton
1938–39

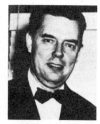
Philip S. Hench
1939–40

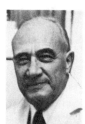
Ralph H. Boots
1940–41

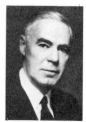
Loring T. Swain
1941–42

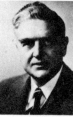
W. Paul Holbrook
1942–45

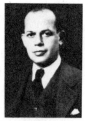
Walter Bauer
1946–47

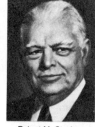
Robert M. Stecher
1947–48
President International League
1953–57

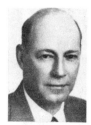
Richard H. Freyberg
1948–49

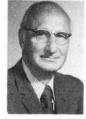
T. Duckett Jones
1949–50

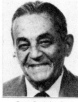
Otto Steinbroker
1950–51

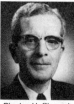
Charles H. Slocumb
1951–52

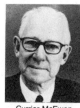
Currier McEwen
1952–53

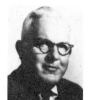
Charles Ragan
1953–54

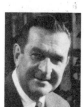
Edward W. Boland
1954–55

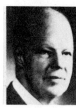
Charles L. Short
1955–56

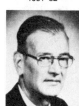
William D. Robinson
1856–57

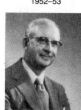
L. Maxwell Lockie
1957–58

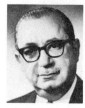
Joseph J. Bunim
1958–59

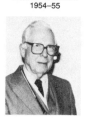
Charley J. Smyth
1959–60

Figure 3-6. Presidents of the American Rheumatism Association, first 25 years.

report was signed by Drs. Ralph Pemberton, President of the International League; Philip S. Hench, President of the American Rheumatism Association; and Loring T. Swaim, Secretary of the American Committee of the International League. This was a sad turn of events and the beginning of the dark war years of the early 1940s.

Efforts to continue the objectives of the American Rheumatism Association became increasingly difficult because of the developing world war. After 1942 no meetings were held until the war ended. Many members and leaders of the ARA served in the Armed Forces. Five army hospitals were designated for care of military personnel who had rheumatic illnesses; three were for patients with rheumatic fever and two, for other forms of rheumatic disease. On the professional staff of these army rheumatism centers were many prominent members of ARA (see Chapter 2). This attention paid to rheumatism in the military and the few civilian centers that continued to operate, although low key, kept interest in rheumatic disease alive in the United States.

An assessment of the campaign against rheumatism in the United States in the 1930s shows that significant progress was made. The 1930s can be called the "Missionary Decade" in rheumatism. Recall that the primary purpose of the American Committee was to arouse interest among physicians and the public in the problems of the rheumatic diseases and to emphasize the need for indepth research leading to better treatment and eventual control of these illnesses. In these early years, the crusade concentrated on recruiting physicians to study rheumatic diseases and to conduct research in this neglected field. From the handful of physicians comprising the American Committee, the American Rheumatism Association grew steadily in membership, until it numbered 226 in 1940 and 260 in 1944. The annual meetings attracted more participants and a larger attendance; the scientific sessions expanded from half-day to full-day meetings. The pathologic and clinical characteristics of the major forms of arthritis became better understood; confusion in terminology was reduced; classification of the rheumatic diseases was improved. Several arthritis research centers were established, and medical colleges began to include arthritis in their curricula. In many medical centers, arthritis clinics were established and staffed mostly by ARA members, thus improving the care of arthritis sufferers. Regional rheumatism societies (professional membership) were formed in large cities. They conducted scientific conferences that supplemented the professional education program begun by the American Committee and expanded by the American Rheumatism Association.

4

Origin of the Arthritis and Rheumatism Foundation

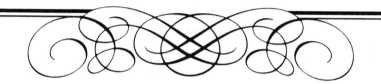

OFFICERS of the American Rheumatism Association elected in 1942 continued in office during the war years. After the war, President Holbrook rallied the ARA Executive Committee to make plans for reactivating the Association. The postwar "reunion meeting" was held in June 1946 in New York City. It was well attended and enthusiasm ran high. Dr. Holbrook delivered a hard-hitting, inspiring president's address, in which he deplored the lack of research in the field of rheumatism. He literally shouted the closing line, which these authors remember as, "So I urge you to return to your homeland, beat the drums, stalk the bushes, light fires, organize local rheumatism societies, establish clinics, and get physicians and the public aroused to work together to lick this monster—arthritis." He recommended that a strong education and research committee be appointed to develop professional and lay education programs, to expand research in the rheumatic diseases, and to explore means of obtaining funds to finance these programs.

The need to raise funds to support the programs of the ARA had been identified before. In 1942 the ARA Executive Committee had discussed plans to organize a campaign to raise funds to support a continuing program of education, research, and patient care, but action was delayed by World War II. How similar this situation was to the delay in progress of the campaign against rheumatism started by van Breemen, which was ground to a halt by World War I!

One of the first official actions of the incoming ARA President in 1946, Dr. Walter Bauer, was to appoint Dr. Holbrook Chairman of a new Education and Research (E and R) Committee and direct him to select the members. The committee was instructed to report results of its studies and make recommendations for implementing programs at the next Executive Committee meeting. Dr. Holbrook appointed a large committee of members from all sections of the United States.

To expedite the Committee's work, Dr. Holbrook designated a subcommittee composed of the New York members and appointed Dr. Richard Freyberg Chairman. This subcommittee met early on and recommended consultation with a professional fundraising firm to plan a continuing campaign for funds to finance the expanding research and education programs in this field.

The New York firm of John Price Jones (JPJ) was consulted because of its extensive experience in conducting fundraising campaigns for other health agencies. John Price Jones recommended that a national voluntary health agency composed of both professional and lay personnel be formed for arthritis and rheumatism, that this agency be separate from the American Rheumatism Association, and that it be a foundation primarily for the purpose of raising funds to support the education and research programs of ARA. JPJ was convinced that if strong lay leadership were obtained for the foundation, success would be assured and the goals would be achieved.

John Price Jones further advised that a national survey be conducted to determine the status of and voids in 1) research into the problems of arthritis and allied conditions, 2) professional and lay education in this medical field, and 3) care of persons suffering from rheumatic diseases. The committee believed the survey should be done with the cooperation and assistance of the National Research Council (NRC) to enhance the credibility and public acceptance of the results. Such a survey was expected to expose the neglect of the rheumatic diseases and justify organization of a voluntary health agency to raise funds for arthritis and rheumatism. Further, the survey would furnish a sound basis with which to plan programs of investigation, education, and patient care in the field of rheumatic diseases.

The Education and Research Committee met twice in New York City to formulate its report to the ARA Executive Committee in June 1947. The report, which summarized the advice from John Price Jones, concluded with these recommendations: 1) that the opinion of the National Research Council be obtained regarding the need at this time for a voluntary health agency to work in the field of rheumatism, 2) if the NRC response were affirmative, that NRC be requested to assist in making the survey advised by JPJ, and 3) that a national voluntary health agency sponsored by ARA be formed without delay.

The Executive Committee endorsed the report and presented it to the ARA membership the following day for approval. Members of ARA voted approval enthusiastically and authorized enactment of the recommendations of the Education and Research Committee. The Committee was authorized to solicit contributions to defray expenses of the NRC survey and to pay for the services of John Price Jones. This ARA action was the spark that led to formation of the *Arthritis and Rheumatism Foundation*.

At this point, the E and R Committee really had its work cut out! John Price Jones was engaged to help organize the Foundation, to assist in obtaining "seed money" and to help recruit lay members. JPJ recommended that the structure of the Foundation be that of a central body with national headquarters and many chapters widely scattered throughout the United States, each working independently in carrying out the Foundation's work but closely coordinated with the national organization.

Several nationally known laypersons interested in arthritis were proposed by JPJ and members of ARA to be directors of the Foundation. Drs. Ralph Boots, Russell Cecil, and Richard Freyberg were appointed to choose someone to serve as Chairman of the Board of Directors of the Foundation. This committee agreed that one person was a "natural" to provide the strong leadership needed of the chairman: Mr. Floyd B. Odlum, Chairman of the Board of Atlas Corporation. Mr. Odlum was prominent in the business and financial world and well known for his ability to provide leadership to struggling, young business organizations. He was intensely interested in a national campaign against rheumatism because he suffered severely from rheumatoid arthritis and deplored the neglect of this serious health problem. When the Chairmanship of the Board of Directors was proposed to him, he was eager to serve but hesitated because he thought his poor health might prevent him from doing a job of excellence, always his goal. After a few months, his health improved, and he agreed to commit himself to the task, at least during the period of organization.

With the help of Mr. Odlum and Mr. Hayden Smith, a prominent New York lawyer who agreed to serve as a director, several other nationally known business and professional men were invited and agreed to become directors. Money to defray organizational expenses was obtained from a few corporations and from several individuals who wished to remain anonymous. All seemed to be in order for the Education and Research Committee to proceed with the formation of the Foundation.

NATIONAL RESEARCH COUNCIL COMES INTO THE PICTURE

A delegation of the ARA met with members of the National Research Council at the American Academy of Sciences in Washington, DC on September 19, 1947. Present at this meeting for ARA were Drs. Walter Bauer, Ralph Boots, Richard Freyberg, T. Duckett Jones, Currier McEwen, and Cornelius Traeger; for the National Academy of Sciences, Dr. A. N. Richards; for the NRC, Drs. Lewis Weed, Chairman of the Division of Medical Sciences, Raymond Werner, Philip Owen, and Hayden Nickolson. Also present was Mr. Harold Weeks of John Price Jones.

As spokesman for the ARA, Dr. Freyberg reviewed the ARA's plans for a fundraising campaign and stated that the Association desired guidance and assistance from NRC, particularly in making the national survey of research, educational, and clinical facilities.

Both Dr. Richards and Dr. Weed felt the time was right for the formation of a national voluntary health agency for arthritis and rheumatism. Dr. Weed advised, as had John Price Jones, that ARA continue as a separate professional organization to be responsible for medical and lay education and research in the field of rheumatic diseases and that a new agency, a Foundation, be formed to collect and disburse funds to finance the ARA programs. The remainder of the meeting was devoted to outlining a plan of procedure.

Dr. Weed advised ARA to request NRC to appoint a continuing committee that, as a first step, would conduct the survey and then recommend the direction of future research. He estimated the survey would cost $15,000.

A summary of the discussion of this meeting was sent to the Chairman of the E and R Committee. The Committee officially requested NRC to appoint a committee to do the survey and recommend research. Funds to defray the expenses were obtained from contributions made by interested laymen and ARA physicians who wished to remain anonymous.

Survey by National Research Council. The Committee appointed by the National Research Council to direct the survey was composed of the following:

Physicians	Medical Discipline
Walter Bauer	Internal Medicine and Arthritis
Robert Elman	Surgery
Richard H. Freyberg	Internal Medicine and Arthritis
Ralph W. Gerard	Physiologist (Neuro-Physiology)
Philip S. Hench	Internal Medicine and Arthritis
C. N. H. Long	Biochemistry and Endocrinology
Colin M. MacLeod	Bacteriology
Karl Meyer	Enzyme Chemistry
Edward S. Rogers	Public Health
Howard A. Rusk	Rehabilitation
Francis O. Schmitt	Biology and Biophysics
Joseph Ney	Executive Secretary

The survey was started immediately. The first task was to prepare a questionnaire to be sent to the deans of all medical schools in the United States inquiring 1) what investigation of arthritis and allied conditions was being conducted, the source of funding, which physicians and scientists were participating, and the expected duration of the research; 2) whether there were hospital beds for patients with rheumatic disease; if so, the number of beds alloted; whether there was an arthritis clinic in that institution; 3) what instruction in rheumatic diseases was given in the medical school; and 4) if funds became available, whether the institution would be interested in conducting research and training clinicians in the rheumatic diseases.

The second part of the Committee's work, that of preparing a long-range program of research in rheumatic diseases, was undertaken in the following manner. Research to be recommended was considered in three categories. The Committee was divided into three subcommittees, one for each category. Dr. Schmitt was appointed Chairman of the subcommittee to recommend research projects in the general understanding of mesenchymal tissue. Dr. Freyberg was designated Chairman of the subcommittee on specific problems of arthritis and rheumatic diseases. Recommendations for research into public health aspects and social, environmental, and economic problems of the rheumatic diseases were to be made by a subcommittee chaired by Dr. Rogers. The results of the survey were combined with the recommendations of the three subcommittees into a preliminary report submitted in November 1948. The final report of the NRC Committee was made to the Arthritis and Rheumatism Foundation in April 1949.

PLANS DRAFTED FOR INCORPORATION OF THE FOUNDATION

While the survey was being conducted, John Price Jones drafted a plan for organization of the Foundation and for conducting its fundraising campaign. To assist in these tasks, several prospective members of the Board of Directors were appointed to the Education and Research Committee: Floyd B. Odlum, Hayden N. Smith, David G. Baird, George L. Harrison, and Cyril H. Jones.

During preparation of the documents for incorporating the Foundation, it was learned that other organizations existed to study arthritis and allied conditions and to solicit funds nationally for research support. One was the National Arthritis Research Foundation, sponsored by B'nai B'rith; Chairman of its Board of Directors was Judge Abraham B. Frey, a prominent St. Louis lawyer. This Foundation was planning a campaign to raise funds to establish an arthritis research center at Levi Memorial Hospital in Hot Springs, Arkansas. Another organization soliciting contributions to support arthritis research was the Detroit

Fund for Crippling Diseases, Inc., started by Dr. Earl Peterman. Two other groups, the American Anti-Arthritis Association, organized in 1945 by the Los Angeles Rheumatism Association, and the District of Columbia Arthritis Foundation in Washington, DC, were planning fundraising campaigns to finance arthritis research.

The Education and Research Committee appreciated the well-intentioned purposes of each of these organizations. However, it felt that several organizations competing nationally for funds for the same purpose would be inefficient and confusing to the public. Accordingly, representatives of the Committee and the National Research Council visited leaders of these other groups to encourage them to continue their efforts but confine fundraising to their localities and join with the ARA in a national campaign. The National Arthritis Research Foundation and the Detroit Fund for Crippling Diseases agreed to confine their efforts to local programs and to fully support the ARA-sponsored national campaign. Judge Frey accepted a directorship in the new Foundation, and the trustees of the Detroit Fund for Crippling Diseases proposed two of their group to be considered as directors of the ARA-sponsored Foundation. The other organizations agreed to support the proposed Foundation. Thus a unity of efforts was accomplished in a national voluntary health agency to fight arthritis.

ESTABLISHMENT OF THE FOUNDATION

The way was then clear for ARA to form a foundation to fight arthritis without competition. In March 1948 a certificate requesting permission for incorporation of the *American Rheumatism Foundation* was filed in the office of the Secretary of State of New York. In this document, the purposes for which the Foundation was to be formed were stated:

> to stimulate and to provide ways and means for the study of research as to, and the collection, dissemination, and application of knowledge concerning the nature and causes, and methods and techniques or the treatment, alleviation, cure, and prevention of arthritis, rheumatic fever and other rheumatic and kindred or contributory ailments; and in order to carry out the foregoing, to solicit and obtain voluntary contributions and receive and administer monies and properties and to expend and use such monies and properties either through itself or through voluntary gifts or grants to other institutions, agencies, groups, corporations and individuals for the furtherance of the purposes hereinabove set forth.
>
> The territory in which its operations are principally to be conducted is in the United States of America.
>
> The principal office of the Corporation is to be located in the Borough of Manhattan, City, County and State of New York.
>
> The number of its Directors shall be not less than five and not more than twenty-five.
>
> The names of the Directors until the first corporate meeting are:

David G. Baird	Montclair, New Jersey
Walter Bauer, MD	Boston, Massachusetts
Ralph H. Boots, MD	New York, New York
Judge Abraham B. Frey	St. Louis, Missouri
Richard H. Freyberg, MD	Scarsdale, New York
George L. Harrison	New York, New York
W. Paul Holbrook, MD	Tucson, Arizona
Cyril H. Jones	Shelburne, Vermont
Floyd B. Odlum	Indio, California
Hayden N. Smith	New York, New York

Charley J. Smyth, MD   Detroit, Michigan
Robert M. Stecher, MD   Cleveland, Ohio
        In witness whereof, we do make, subscribe and acknowledge this Certificate
this 3rd day of March, 1948.

(Signed)
Richard H. Freyberg
George L. Harrison
W. Paul Holbrook
Cyril H. Jones
Hayden N. Smith

FIRST MEETING OF THE DIRECTORS OF THE NEW FOUNDATION

The organizational meeting of Incorporators and Directors of the *American Rheumatism Foundation* was held in the boardroom of the College of Medicine of New York University on May 6, 1948. The meeting was attended by six of the 12 directors and, by invitation, Mr. Harold Weeks of John Price Jones. Mr. Hayden Smith was chosen Chairman of the meeting.

A constitution and bylaws were adopted. The persons named as Directors in the Certificate of Incorporation were elected Directors of the Foundation (Figure 4-1).

Officers elected to serve until the first special meeting were: Floyd B. Odlum, Chairman of the Board; Dr. W. Paul Holbrook, President; Cyril H. Jones, Vice Chairman of the Board and Vice President; Hayden N. Smith, Treasurer; Dr. Charley J. Smyth, Secretary; Dr. Charles A. Ragan, Jr., Assistant Secretary; Dr. John G. Kuhns, Assistant Treasurer.

An Executive Committee was designated to consist of: Floyd B. Odlum, Dr. W. Paul Holbrook, Cyril H. Jones, David C. Baird, and Drs. Richard H. Freyberg, Charley J. Smyth, and Robert M. Stecher. A Financial and Investment Committee was created.

The Directors expressed their gratitude to the persons who contributed funds for the NRC survey. A resolution was adopted expressing appreciation to the organizations that joined with the American Rheumatism Association to establish the Foundation. Temporary offices were established at 150 Nassau Street, New York City or at the office of the Chairman of the Board, 33 Pine Street, New York.

So was born the American Rheumatism Foundation!

1948—A BUSY YEAR

This new organization had given itself an imposing agenda with a close deadline—the first fundraising campaign was to begin in the fall. So much was to be done that seven special meetings of the Directors were called in 1948, one each month from June through December. The meetings were held either in Mr. Odlum's office or home and focused on completing the organization and internal structure of the Foundation, publicizing its existence and purposes, chartering chapters, organizing the first fundraising campaign, and starting its medical program.

Organizational Matters. Officers elected to serve until the first annual meeting were: Floyd B. Odlum, Chairman of the Board of Directors and the Executive Committee; W. Paul Holbrook, MD, President; Cyril H. Jones, Vice Chairman of the Board and Vice President; Hayden N. Smith, Secretary; James G. Blaine, Treasurer; Charles A. Ragan, Jr., MD, Assistant Secretary; and J. Frank Morris, Assistant Treasurer.

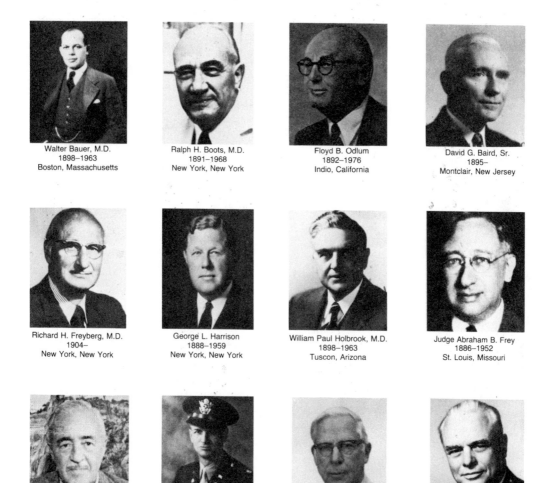

Figure 4-1. Founding directors of the Arthritis and Rheumatism Foundation.

Between meetings of the Board of Directors, the Board's powers and duties would be conducted by an Executive Committee consisting of the Chairman of the Board of Directors, the President of the Foundation, and other members of the Board of Directors designated by the Board. The chairman of the Executive Committee would be the Chief Executive Officer of the Foundation.

A Medical Committee was appointed to consist of the following physicians (subject to acceptance): Drs. Guy Caldwell, New Orleans; Russell L. Cecil, New York; Robley Evans, Boston; Morris Fishbein, Chicago; Philip S. Hench, Rochester, Minnesota; Albert C. Ivy, Chicago; Currier McEwen, New York; Karl Meyer, San Francisco; Walter Palmer, New York; John Romano, Cincinnati; and Howard Rusk, New York. The name of the Committee was changed to the *Medical and Scientific Committee* (M and S Committee).

Table 4-1. Arthritis and Rheumatism Foundation chapters chartered in 1948

Name of Chapter	Date Charter Issued	Territory Covered
Michigan	September 9, 1948	State of Michigan
New York	October 18, 1948	State of New York
Arkansas	October 29, 1948	State of Arkansas
Eastern Pennsylvania	October 29, 1948	Eastern Pennsylvania
Western Pennsylvania	October 29, 1948	Western Pennsylvania
Southwest	November 4, 1948	States of Arizona, New Mexico, Nevada, Utah, Western Texas
District of Columbia	November 8, 1948	Metropolitan District of Columbia
New England	December 1, 1948	States of Maine, Massachusetts, New Hampshire, Vermont, Rhode Island, Connecticut
Southern California	December 13, 1948	Counties of San Luis Obispo, Kern, San Bernardino, Santa Barbara, Ventura, Los Angeles, Riverside, Orange, San Diego
Northern California	December 13, 1948	Counties of Monterey, Kings, Tulare, Indio, and all counties north of these in California
Maryland	December 20, 1948	State of Maryland

Dr. Richard Freyberg was appointed Temporary Chairman of the M and S Committee and directed to convene the Committee as soon as possible. He was to assist the Committee in its organization and in the development of a medical program and search for a Medical Director.

Bylaws of the Foundation were changed to allow 50 directors. Through the year, 15 additional directors were elected.

The Chairman expressed concern that the name of the Foundation did not include the word *arthritis*; he felt more people were aware of the serious impact of arthritis than of other forms of rheumatism. In compliance with his request, the name of the Foundation was changed to the *Arthritis and Rheumatism Foundation.*

Chapters Chartered. In 1948 charters were granted for the formation of 11 local or regional chapters of the Foundation. The dates the charters were issued and the territory each covered are shown in Table 4-1. A form for a constitution and bylaws to govern the activities of each chapter was approved.

Publicity Regarding the Foundation. The President was requested to inform the medical profession and the public about the formation of the new voluntary health agency for arthritis. His announcement was published in the medical news section of the July 24th issue of the *Journal of the American Medical Association (JAMA).* Dr. Holbrook outlined the objectives of the Foundation as set forth in the Articles of Incorporation. He stated that the first annual fundraising campaign was to be launched in late 1948; the support of the medical and allied professions was requested. The same issue of *JAMA* included an editorial by Dr. Morris Fishbein, the Journal's Editor and a member of the Medical and Scientific Committee, urging support of the medical profession and the public for the Foundation. Announcements and editorials such as these appeared in professional specialty periodicals and in state and county medical society journals and were very effective in gaining acceptance and cooperation of the medical profession. For the lay public, articles announcing the formation of the Foundation and explaining its purpose and objectives were published in newspapers and popular magazines.

The First Fundraising Campaign. The Foundation scheduled the first campaign to start in the fall of 1948. John Price Jones estimated the expense of conducting the drive to be $150,000 to $200,000 and advised that these funds should be raised as soon as possible. The Officers and Directors of the Foundation appealed to each other, to friends, to philanthropic foundations, and to industry and by August had received sufficient contributions to defray the expenses of the fundraising drive. It was decided to launch the campaign in November with a goal of $2 million. Bob Hope agreed to be Honorary Chairman and LeRoy Campbell, Director, was chosen to be the active campaign Chairman.

The campaign got off to a good start. Announcements of the upcoming drive appeared in news media and professional and lay journals. During the campaign, appeals to the public for contributions were made on radio, television, and widely scattered posters.

FOUNDATION SUPPORTS THE SEVENTH INTERNATIONAL CONGRESS

The American Rheumatism Association delegated a committee to inform the Directors of the Foundation that the Seventh International Congress on Rheumatic Diseases sponsored by the International League Against Rheumatism would be held in New York City in 1949, with ARA acting as host. The Committee was also to request financial support from the Foundation for the Congress. The Directors received this information enthusiastically; they agreed the event should inaugurate its professional education program and resolved that 5% of the money raised in the upcoming fundraising campaign, but not more than $50,000, be allocated to support the Congress. Because this appropriation was to be made from funds not yet in hand, Charles B. Wrightsman, a Director, generously offered to contribute the difference required to make up the $50,000 should campaign funds be insufficient. This grant, the first made by the Foundation, assured the expenses of the Seventh International Congress would be met.

In sum, what a year of accomplishment! The Foundation had been formed and was in business; charters had been issued for 11 chapters; the first national fundraising campaign for arthritis and rheumatism had been launched, and the Foundation had begun its professional education program by granting funds to support the Seventh International Congress on Rheumatic Diseases.

The successful organization of the Arthritis and Rheumatism Foundation is attributable largely to the energy and dedication of one man—Floyd B. Odlum. If the E and R Committee of ARA put it all together, Mr. Odlum kept it all together through this difficult year, and during a time when he was ill with rheumatoid arthritis.

5

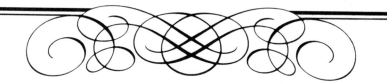

Foundation Activities 1949-1950

AT the beginning of 1949 organization of the staff of the Arthritis and Rheumatism Foundation was started. Mr. Thomas Freeman, appointed on January 1 to be Executive Director, was the first salaried staff member. Experience he had gained working with other voluntary health agencies proved valuable to the new Foundation. The services of John Price Jones were continued on a limited basis to assist in organizing chapters and in fundraising. Mr. Norman Winter was appointed to serve as Director of Public Relations.

On January 5, 1949 the Medical and Scientific Committee of the Arthritis and Rheumatism Foundation convened in New York City to organize a medical program for the Foundation. New appointees to the Committee were: Drs. Richard Freyberg, T. Duckett Jones, Colin M. MacLeod, and Hugh McCulloch. Dr. Russell Cecil was elected Chairman for the first year and Dr. Freyberg, Vice Chairman. Until a medical director was appointed, the Chairman of the Medical and Scientific Committee was designated to act in this capacity; Dr. Cecil thus became the first "acting" Medical Director of the Foundation.

A subcommittee was appointed to handle release of material to the news media; Dr. Morris Fishbein was named Chairman. Another subcommittee to establish standards for clinical and educational programs was appointed, with Dr. Currier McEwen as Chairman. The Medical and Scientific Committee unanimously agreed that the top priority in the Foundation's medical program in the early years should be to foster training of more investigators and clinicians in rheumatic diseases. This priority led to the early development of the Foundation's fellowship program. The Committee also endorsed the decision of the Directors that the Foundation would support the Seventh International Congress on Rheumatic Diseases.

FIRST ANNUAL MEETING OF THE FOUNDATION

At the first annual meeting of the Foundation, held in New York City in May 1949, just before the Seventh International Congress, the Chairman reported:

> Charters were issued for two new chapters in the early months of 1949....
>
> In the fund raising drive, a total of $266,458 had been received. Although far from the goal set, it is considered satisfactory realizing that most of the chapters were newly organized and not geared to efficient operation.
>
> The report of the NRC survey was received in April. The questionnaire revealed that a total of 222 research projects were being conducted in 51 institutions in the U.S. All of the 70 institutions contacted in the survey declared themselves desirous of doing more research and 65 were interested and able to train additional research personnel pending financial aid. The NRC report contained extensive recommendations for research considered likely to be profitable in the field of rheumatism.
>
> In supporting the Seventh International Congress on Rheumatic Diseases, the Foundation inaugurated its professional educational program.
>
> In conclusion it may be said with confidence that a good start has been made in accomplishing the program of the Foundation and that we can look to the future with a feeling of confidence that a comprehensive attack can be made to conquer rheumatic diseases. There are good reasons for optimism.

THE SEVENTH INTERNATIONAL CONGRESS ON RHEUMATIC DISEASES

A year before the Seventh International Congress was to be held, the American Rheumatism Association committed itself to act as host and agreed to accept responsibility for all preparations for the meetings. The Congress was to be held in New York City, May 30 through June 3, 1949. A large Planning Committee was appointed with Dr. Philip Hench as Chairman. On this Committee were the President of le Ligue International contre le Rhumatisme, Dr. Ralph Pemberton, the President of the ARA, and many members of the ARA Executive Committee and the Medical and Scientific Committee of the Foundation. The Planning Committee met several times in 1948 and 1949 to organize the scientific and social programs. It soon became evident the task was too large for an all-volunteer committee, so it was decided to employ professional assistance.

The Committee was fortunate to be able to engage the services of Mr. Robert Potter, an accomplished science writer, to act as Executive Secretary and Coordinator of Plans for the Congress. Working out of the office of the Foundation, he efficiently carried out the policies of the Planning Committee. His experience in science writing proved invaluable, especially in arranging press coverage before and during the Congress and in assisting the ARA committee in editing the *Proceedings* of the Congress in a monograph published in 1952 (113). He became so interested in the problems of arthritis and rheumatism that he stayed on with the ARA as Executive Secretary.

The scientific program of the Seventh International Congress included reports and discussions of topics then of interest in rheumatic diseases. It was a full program, for this Congress served as a combined meeting of the International League and the annual session of ARA. Plenary sessions, symposia, and panel discussions on topics of special interest were held daily in the Waldorf Astoria Hotel, and many live clinics and workshops were held in the medical schools and teaching hospitals in the New York area. All meetings were well attended; in addition to more than 500 physicians and scientists who registered for the

Congress, a large number of practicing physicians and faculty members of regional medical schools were invited to attend.

The highlight of the scientific program was the presentation by Drs. Hench, Kendall, Slocumb, and Polley of the remarkable effects of cortisone and ACTH on patients with rheumatoid arthritis. Although a preliminary report of this important discovery had been presented at a meeting of the staff of the Mayo Clinic on April 20, 1949 (62), the presentation at the Seventh International Congress was the first on cortisone given at an international meeting of physicians and scientists whose principal interest was the study and treatment of rheumatic disease. The presentation was dramatic! Superb cinema and lantern slides illustrated the clinical effects of cortisone. The report made a great impression on all who heard and saw it.

Excellent press coverage by well-informed science writers gave worldwide exposure to the events of the Congress. The mere fact that an International Congress on Rheumatic Diseases was held in New York in 1949 and was so well attended by an international group of investigators and practicing physicians was evidence that, at last, rheumatic diseases were capturing widespread attention of the medical profession and that progress was being made in the United States in the knowledge and treatment of these diseases.

The events of the Congress had far-reaching benefits. The scientific reports presented at the Congress, capped by the cortisone story, gave those suffering from arthritis new hope and reason to dispel the gloom that had prevailed. To the professionals already studying rheumatism, the reports were very exciting and further stimulated interest in their studies. Young investigators and clinicians were attracted to the study of rheumatism.

One sad note rang through the Seventh International Congress. Dr. Ralph Pemberton, who was President of the International League from 1939 through the war years, who headed the planning committee for the Congress that was to be held in New York, Boston, and Philadelphia in 1940 (but was later cancelled because of the impending war), who then worked diligently with the planning committee for the 1949 Congress, and who was the one most responsible for the formation of the ARA, was unable to attend because of the illness that caused his death shortly after the Congress—a great loss to the fight against rheumatism in the United States and throughout the world!

REORGANIZATION OF LE LIGUE INTERNATIONAL CONTRE LE RHUMATISME

Eleven years had elapsed since the last International Congress on Rheumatic Diseases. Activities of the International League had been suspended during the war years and the postwar recovery period. However, the officers elected at the 1938 congress in London had continued to serve throughout these years. The League's governing body met in New York a few days before the 1949 Congress to revise the constitution and bylaws and change the structure of the organization.

Several events had occurred in the 1940s that made it necessary to restructure the League. During the early war years, Dr. Anibal Ruiz-Moreno of Buenos Aires, President of the National Rheumatism Society of Argentina, had met with leaders of several other national rheumatism societies in North and South America and recommended that a continental league of these societies be formed. In the United States Dr. Ruiz-Moreno discussed this proposition with Drs. Ralph Pemberton, Loring Swaim, and others who were enthusiastically in favor of the idea. After discussion with officers of the International League

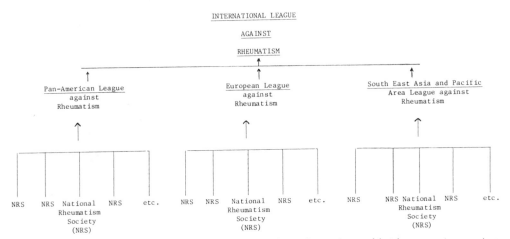

Figure 5-1. Schematic representation of the medical profession's worldwide campaign against rheumatism.

Against Rheumatism, who also approved of an American continental league, it was agreed that Drs. Ruiz-Moreno, Pemberton, and Swaim would act as a committee to organize the league. The task was completed in May 1944, and announcement of the formation of the *Pan-American League for the Study and Control of Rheumatic Diseases* (later known as Pan-American League Against Rheumatism, or PANLAR) was made in July 1944. This first continental league comprised the rheumatism societies of Argentina, Brazil, Canada, Chile, Mexico, Paraguay, Peru, United States, and Uruguay.

In September 1947 the rheumatism societies in Europe joined to form the European League Against Rheumatism (EULAR). Before 1949 le Ligue International was made up of these European societies and the societies in the Americas. After its reorganization in New York, le Ligue International (the International League Against Rheumatism, or ILAR) was composed of the continental leagues and the few national rheumatism societies outside the province of the Pan-American and European Leagues.

In September 1963 the national rheumatism societies in the countries of Southeast Asia and the Pacific area joined to form the *Southeast Asia and Pacific Area League Against Rheumatism* (SEAPAL). ILAR thus became made up of the three multinational leagues PANLAR, EULAR, and SEAPAL, with financial support coming from all three leagues (Figure 5-1).

On the day before the 1949 opening of the Seventh International Congress, delegates to the governing bodies of the Pan-American and European Leagues met to update the bylaws and plan future activities. PANLAR and EULAR each decided to hold a continental congress on rheumatic diseases in the years between ILAR-sponsored international congresses, which would be held every four years. After SEAPAL was formed, it was decided that between international congresses, a league-sponsored congress would be held every year. These continental congresses would be sponsored in rotation by EULAR, PANLAR, and SEAPAL.

THE FOUNDATION GOES INTO HIGH GEAR

In 1949 much was done to strengthen the Arthritis and Rheumatism Foundation. The appointment of Thomas Freeman as Executive Director improved coordination of the

Foundation's program. New chapters were formed. Existing chapters were strengthened by the addition of laymen to their Boards of Directors and of physicians, mostly members of ARA-affiliated regional rheumatic societies, on the Medical and Scientific Committees. The Foundation's national headquarters supplied the chapters with guidelines for conducting public education forums and fundraising drives.

General Lucius Clay, USA retired, accepted the position of Campaign Chairman for the second national fundraising drive. General Clay appointed a large "Sponsors Committee" of 77 leaders in business and public affairs from all parts of the nation to assist him in organizing the campaign scheduled to begin in the fall of 1949. To "kick off" the campaign, dinner parties were held in cities in areas with active chapters. Prominent laymen and physicians spoke at these gatherings, appealing for contributions to support the programs of the Foundation. In New York City, the kick-off dinner was staged by the New York Chapter together with the Foundation headquarters. National and chapter officers participated in the program. In Boston, seminars for physicians and public meetings were held in which leaders in rheumatism research and officers of the New England Chapter participated. Such fundraising activities provided excellent publicity for the campaign. Contributions in the second drive for funds amounted to $650,000, more than double the amount raised in the first campaign.

In 1950 the Foundation established its national headquarters at 535 Fifth Avenue, New York City. Dr. Gideon K. DeForest was appointed Medical Director. Dr. DeForest had been active in research on rheumatic diseases while serving on the faculty of Yale Medical School. He was leader of the group that formed the Connecticut Chapter of the Foundation. His expertise was an important factor in getting the Foundation's medical program into full swing.

FELLOWSHIP PROGRAM

The Fellowship Program was launched in 1950 in response to the recommendations of the National Research Council. The Council had considered the research projects in arthritis currently under way to be "of small extent, inadequately staffed and inadequately supported, with a large portion of available funds going into rheumatic fever research" (112).

In the entire United States, only $300,000 was being spent on chronic arthritis research, the Council reported, adding that more than three times that amount was needed annually to adequately address the problem. In 1949 it was estimated that 7.5 million people had some type of rheumatic disease. At the conclusion of its 1949 report, the Council stressed that all research institutions were in dire need of more funds and that the first priority in the research program should be the training of competent investigators.

With its problems clearly delineated, the Medical and Scientific Committee had to answer a number of policy questions: What type of research should be supported? Should funds be allocated as grants-in-aid for specific projects or given as direct grants to individual investigators?

The Committee decided that available funds should be directed into basic research rather than into clinical studies on specific rheumatic diseases. The Committee members further determined that in the evaluation of a fellowship application, primary consideration should be given to the applicant's potential as a productive, independent investigator, rather than to the specific nature of the proposed research project. Although the Foundation itself was still in its early stages of formation, the Committee recommended that funds be allocated at once. Announcements of the fellowships to be awarded by the Foundation were sent out early in 1950 to all medical schools in the United States. Twenty-two young investigators responded, and a newly formed Fellowship Committee processed the applications.

The first awardees of the fellowship competition were Max W. Biggs, MD, PhD; Felix DeMartini, MD; Ralph Jessar, MD; George Cytroen, MD; William P. Deiss, Jr., MD, Myron Usdin, PhD; Morris Ziff, MD, PhD. Each recipient received approximately $5,000 for one year's work.

THE PIVOTAL YEARS

In June 1950 the Honorable Robert P. Patterson, former Secretary of War, accepted the presidency of the Arthritis and Rheumatism Foundation, succeeding Dr. Paul Holbrook. Judge Patterson brought much prestige to the Foundation.

So many important events in the campaign against rheumatism occurred in 1948, 1949, and 1950 that these years are considered pivotal in the campaign. During these years arthritis and rheumatism became recognized as a major health problem deserving public and federal government support. Major events were:

1948   The public joined with the medical profession to form the Arthritis and Rheumatism Foundation, to support a national voluntary health agency, to support research and education in rheumatic diseases.

The "LE" cell was discovered (58), and the significance of the agglutination reaction of sensitized sheep cells involving the "rheumatoid factor" was recognized (130).

1949   Cortisone and ACTH were shown to have profound effects on inflammatory arthritis.

More than 500 physicians from all parts of the world convened in a week-long forum, the Seventh International Congress on Rheumatic Diseases, to present and discuss reports of investigations of problems of rheumatism, topped by the cortisone story, giving worldwide exposure to the campaign against rheumatism.

A bill was introduced in the U.S. Congress to support arthritis research with federal funds, which led to legislation in the following year.

1950   The Omnibus Medical Research Act was passed by Congress and signed into law by President Truman, establishing the National Institute of Arthritis and Metabolic Diseases within the National Institutes of Health and authorizing the appointment of the National Advisory Arthritis and Metabolic Diseases Council.

Drs. Hench, Kendall, and Reichstein were awarded the Nobel Prize in Medicine and Physiology for their work with cortisone and corticotrophin.

In these eventful years, research on arthritis and rheumatism emerged from a state of confusion and bewilderment to become more organized, logical, and scientific.

In this transition, the role of cortisone cannot be overestimated. The cortisone story was an event that demonstrated that research could be expected to solve at least some of the many puzzling problems of arthritis. It opened gates to a vast fertile field of arthritis research, which attracted many young investigators. It showed the broad scope of the rheumatic diseases, embracing many disciplines of medicine, endocrinology, metabolism, inflammation, allergy, immunology, and others.

Yes, the events of 1948 through 1950 elevated the study of arthritis and rheumatism to a higher level in the United States. The speciality became dignified by the name *rheumatology*; the physicians engaged in this field were called "rheumatologists," a name not commonly used before 1950. In these mid-century years, rheumatology emerged as a flourishing medical specialty.

6

Origin of the National Institute of Arthritis and Metabolic Diseases

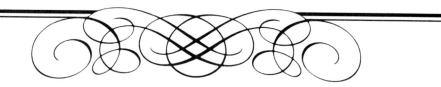

THE crusade for more research in arthritis and rheumatism in the United States took on increased momentum during the 1940s, especially in the postwar years. The United States Public Health Service issued several reports describing the magnitude and importance of rheumatic diseases as a major public health problem. The survey of the National Research Council (NRC) revealed the scant research being conducted and stressed the need for more investigation and facilities to care for patients suffering from arthritis. Armed with the facts in the NRC report, the Public Health Service, under the leadership of Leonard Scheele, MD, Surgeon General, called for government support of research in arthritis and rheumatism. Because government support could be provided only by legislative action, the Public Health Service vigorously pushed for Congressional action.

Working behind the scenes were an increasing number of concerned physicians and health-minded laypersons, pressuring Congress to legislate support for intensified investigation of arthritis and rheumatism. Prominent among the lay group were Mr. and Mrs. Albert Lasker, who, acting individually and through the Lasker Foundation they had formed to foster medical research, assisted substantially in gaining the support of leaders in Congress, notably Senator Lister Hill (Democrat) of Alabama (Figure 6-1) and Representative John Fogerty (Democrat) of Rhode Island, Chairman of the Senate and House Committees on Health (Figure 6-2). The citizen pressure on Congress was greatly intensified by the newly formed national voluntary health agency, the Arthritis and Rheumatism Foundation.

In reaction to these pressures, a bill was introduced in Congress in January 1949 to:

> amend the Public Health Service Act to support research and training in diseases of arthritis and rheumatism, and to aid States in the development of community programs for the control of these diseases, and for other purposes.

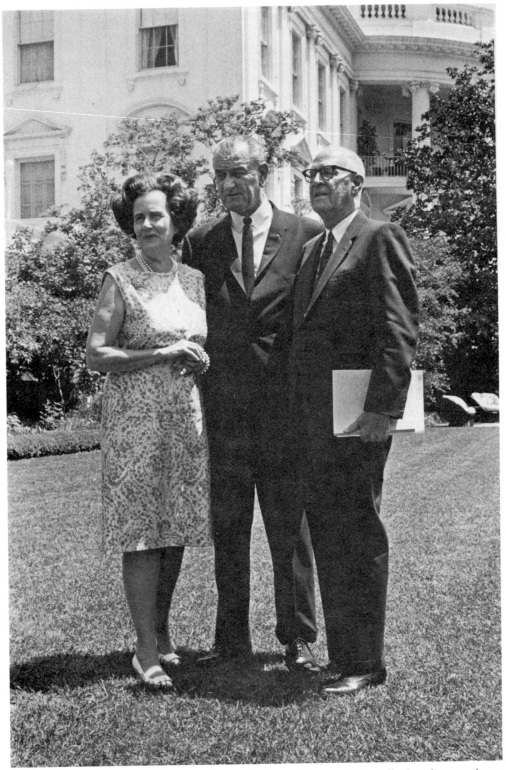

Figure 6-1. President Lyndon Johnson with Mary Lasker and Senator Lister Hill. This photograph was taken in 1968, 20 years after the passage of the Arthritis and Rheumatism Act, which was actually signed into law by President Truman.

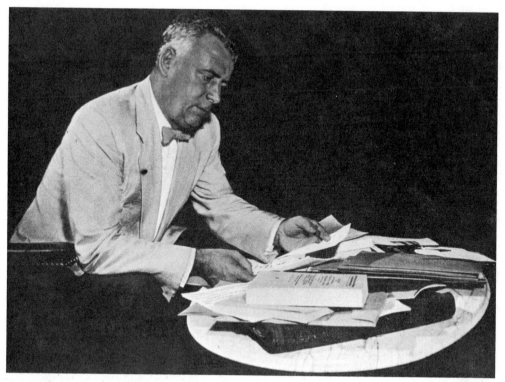

Figure 6-2. Representative John Fogerty, who was instrumental in the passage of the Omnibus Medical Research Act.

Be it enacted by the Senate and House of Representatives of the United States of America in Congress assembled that the Act may be cited as the *National Arthritis and Rheumatism Act.*

The purpose of this Act is to improve the health of the people of the United States through the conduct of researches, investigations, experiments, and demonstrations relating to the cause, prevention, and methods of diagnosis and treatment of diseases; assist and foster such researches and other activities by public and private agencies, and promote the coordination of all such researches and activities and the useful application of their results; provide research and clinical fellowships and training in medical schools in matters relating to arthritis and rheumatism, including refresher courses for physicians, and develop an information center, and assist States and other agencies in the use of, the most effective methods of prevention, diagnosis, and treatment of arthritis and rheumatism, and the rehabilitation of those who have been victims of these diseases, who have been left with residual deformities.

The bill called for the establishment of a *National Arthritis and Rheumatism Institute* in the Public Health Service and for the appointment of a National Advisory Arthritis and Rheumatism Council to assist the Surgeon General in carrying out the purposes of the proposed act.

Hearings before the Senate Subcommittee on Health (of the Committee on Labor and Public Welfare) on the National Arthritis and Rheumatism Bill were held May 9, 1949.

Testimony in support of this bill was given by six witnesses: Drs. Paul Holbrook, President of the Arthritis and Rheumatism Foundation, and Robert M. Stecher, President of ARA, Mr. J. H. McLaurin, Mr. Ralph B. Rogers, and Mr. Frank E. Mandel, all Directors of the Foundation, and Dr. Russell L. Cecil, acting Medical Director of the Foundation. A letter from Floyd B. Odlum, Chairman of the Foundation's Board of Directors was read, urging favorable consideration of the bill.

These witnesses presented forceful testimony. They emphasized the high prevalence of rheumatic diseases in the United States, the suffering, disability, and crippling caused by these conditions, the negative effect on industry because of absenteeism due to these diseases, and the significant economic burden resulting from lost wages and the costs of treatment. The story of cortisone, which broke only two months before the hearing, was used to justify optimism that federal support of research in arthritis and rheumatism would pay off by improving the health of the nation.

However, a snag was encountered that deferred action on the bill at this time. At the hearing, a letter from the Federal Security Agency* was read that stated that many projects relating to arthritis and rheumatism were being conducted in existing Institutes within the National Institutes of Health, especially the Experimental Biology and Medicine Institution. If a new Institute of Arthritis and Rheumatism were added, expensive overlapping and duplication would result. The letter also enumerated other faults with the bill and concluded with, "For the reasons discussed, while in full accord with the basic objectives of the bill, we cannot recommend its favorable consideration." This negative position made changes in the bill necessary.

To avoid the duplication that would result from two institutes in NIH conducting research in rheumatic diseases, a plan was devised to merge the Experimental Biology and Medicine Institute with a new Institute to be called the *National Institute of Arthritis and Metabolic Diseases*. While these changes were being made to the bill, other health bills appeared in Congress, proposing support for research in other fields of medicine. Eventually, all of the health bills were combined into one, the *Omnibus Medical Research Act*, which Congress passed and President Truman signed into law on August 15, 1950. This Act authorized the establishment of the *National Institute of Arthritis and Metabolic Diseases* (NIAMD) in the Public Health Service and the appointment of the National Advisory Arthritis and Metabolic Diseases Council.

The Act specified that the Council include the Surgeons General of the Public Health Service, Army, and Navy, the Chief Medical Officer of the Veterans Administration, and the Chief of the Department of Vocational Rehabilitation, or their representatives, as ex officio members. Twelve members would be appointed to the Council from the fundamental sciences, medical sciences, education, or public affairs; six of the 12 were to be selected from medical or scientific authorities in rheumatic and metabolic diseases. The appointed members of the first council (Figure 6-3) were: *nonmedical*—Mrs. Elinor R. Heller, educator; Dr. Weston Howland, educator; Mr. LeRoy Martin, public affairs; Mr. Floyd Odlum, businessman and Chairman, Board of Directors of the Arthritis and Rheumatism Foundation; Dr. Clyde E. Wildman, educator; *medical*—Drs. Richard H. Freyberg, Philip S. Hench,

---

* The Federal Security Agency, formed in 1935 to administer the Social Security Act, was the forerunner of the Department of Health, Education and Welfare, and later the Department of Health and Human Services. The Public Health Service, including the National Institutes of Health, was transferred to the Federal Security Agency in 1939.

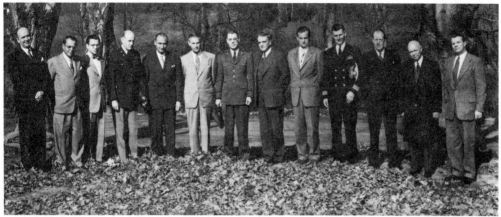

Figure 6-3. First meeting of the National Advisory Arthritis and Metabolic Diseases Council, November 15, 1950, Bethesda, Maryland. From left to right: Dr. William H. Sebrell, Jr., Director of NIAMD, Dr. John A. Reed; Dr. Maxwell Wintrobe; Col. Paul S. Fancher, Alternate, Department of Defense; Dr. Richard Freyberg; Dr. Cecil J. Watson; Lt. Col. William D. Preston, Medical Corps, United States Air Force; Dr. Paul Holbrook; Dr. Alfred H. Lawton, Veterans Administration; Cdr. J. S. Cowan, Medical Corps, United States Navy; Mr. Weston Howland; Mr. Clyde E. Wildman, President, DePauw University; Dr. Floyd S. Doft, Associate Director, NIAMD.

Paul Holbrook, rheumatology; John A. Reed, metabolism; Cecil J. Watson, internal medicine; and Maxwell M. Wintrobe, hematology. The Council first met on November 15, 1950 and approved the first grants in support of research.

On November 22, 1950, in accordance with the Omnibus Medical Research Act, the National Institute of Arthritis and Metabolic Diseases was officially established by Surgeon General Scheele. Dr. W. H. Sebrell, Jr., who had been director of the Experimental Biology and Medicine Institute, was named Director of NIAMD until the new Director could be appointed early in 1951.

The NIAMD was set up to conduct, foster, and support basic and clinical research into arthritis and connective tissue diseases, skin diseases, diseases of bone and muscles, diabetes and other metabolic diseases, and endocrine disorders. The Institute would immediately begin an intramural program of basic studies related to rheumatic, endocrinologic, and metabolic diseases in the laboratories of the Experimental Biology and Medicine Institute. This research would be moved to a new Clinical Center once construction was completed, at which time clinical investigations would begin. NIAMD would also have an extramural program to support basic and clinical research through investigator-initiated research grants, project and center grants, and through career development and training awards. The Council would be concerned mainly with the extramural program.

7

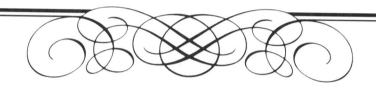

Growth and Contributions of the American Rheumatism Association

AFTER being waged alone by the American Rheumatism Association for 20 years, the United States campaign against rheumatism began to accelerate once the Arthritis and Rheumatism Foundation and the National Institute of Arthritis and Metabolic Diseases came on the scene and provided much-needed financial support. American rheumatology became a fast-growing medical specialty. Recall that the purposes and objectives of all three anti-rheumatism organizations were and are the same, to foster research and education in the field of rheumatism, to provide better treatment, and eventually to bring these diseases under control. Although the three agencies work together in close harmony, each has a different role, so this chapter and the next three will trace the major accomplishments of each, along with those of the Arthritis Health Professions Association (AHPA), which emerged later. Blended together, the achievements of the ARA, the AHPA, the Arthritis and Rheumatism Foundation, and NIAMD account for the progress of American rheumatology since the late 1940s.

Two major functions of the ARA are to encourage and pursue research in the rheumatic diseases and to disseminate the knowledge gained to the medical profession. Committees of the Association have developed classifications and diagnostic criteria for rheumatic diseases that have made clinical studies more useful and comparable with each other. Some committees have also conducted multicenter evaluations of therapeutic measures. The bulk of research by ARA members, however, has been planned and carried out individually in the members' own institutions. The dissemination of knowledge gained through research is accomplished through two channels: scientific meetings at which reports of laboratory and clinical research are presented and discussed and publication of educational literature. Another function of the ARA professional education program is to provide physicians responsible for patient care with the best means of identifying and treating the rheumatic diseases, with the ultimate goal being full control.

GROWTH OF SCIENTIFIC MEETINGS

From the time of its origin, the ARA has held annual scientific meetings, except during the world war years. The nature of the early meetings was reviewed in Chapter 3. The amount of rheumatic disease research rapidly increased with the sharp rise in manpower resulting from the Foundation's fellowship program, with the fellowships, training programs, and research grants of NIAMD, and with the increased number of clinical research centers made possible by the Foundation and the Program-Project grants of NIAMD (see Chapter 10). This abundance of research made it necessary to lengthen the annual meetings and to hold interim meetings. In addition, workshops and seminars on subjects of special interest and review courses were added to the scientific program of the annual meetings. Consequently, the ARA meetings changed considerably since the late 1940s (125).

The first meeting of ARA in 1934 was a one-day session in which 11 papers were presented. In the years until the hiatus of meetings because of World War II, the annual one-day sessions allowed presentation of 10 or 12 papers. When annual meetings resumed after the war, they were lengthened to one and a half, and soon to two-day sessions. The programs became crowded with increasing numbers of presentations, up to 36 by 1954, when interim sessions were introduced. The interim sessions began as one-day meetings, became one and a half, and then two-day sessions. They were held annually in December. The first 10 took place in the Clinical Center of NIH in Bethesda but were held each year after 1965 in a different part of the country.

Even with two meetings a year, so many excellent papers were submitted for the programs that concurrent sessions had to be held during the annual meetings. Beginning in 1963 workshops were added, and soon afterward clinical seminars became part of the program. After the Allied Health Professionals (AHP) section was formed in 1965, annual meetings of AHP were held in conjunction with the annual ARA meetings. In 1976 an innovation was the introduction of poster sessions. Still the number of presentations has continued to grow (Figure 7-1).

The program of the 47th Annual Meeting held in San Antonio in 1983 points up vividly the tremendous growth of the meetings. This three-and-a-half-day meeting included 172 podium papers in four plenary sessions and nineteen concurrent sessions, four workshops covering highly technical scientific subjects, and eight clinical seminars on problems commonly encountered in rheumatologic practice. Poster sessions were held on three days, in which there were 235 presentations. Scientific and commercial exhibits were displayed over three days. Study groups met informally one evening. In all, 442 scientific presentations were made. What a contrast to the situation in 1938 when Dr. McEwen, Chairman of the Program Committee, received so few papers that he wrote to colleagues across the country soliciting more in order to fill a one-day program!

Interim sessions were discontinued in 1972 and replaced the following year with regional winter meetings held annually in different parts of the nation. These meetings quickly became popular. The ARA members are currently organized into four regional groups, the Northeast, Southeast, Central, and Western United States, each having its own officers and committees for conducting the regional winter meetings. The national office helps organize these regional meetings, which consist primarily of papers presented by ARA members of the region. The growth of the scientific programs and the proliferation of ARA annual and regional meetings reflect the progress of rheumatology since 1950.

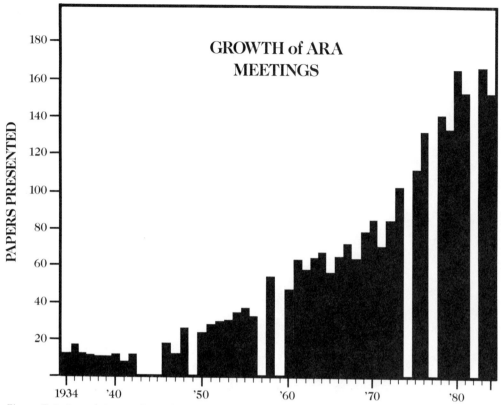

Figure 7-1. Growth in number of podium presentations made at ARA meetings. Years with no data indicate international or continental meetings except for the war years.

GROWTH OF MEMBERSHIP

When the ARA was formed in 1934, 104 physicians were elected as charter members. During the first decade, the membership grew to 272. There was a spurt in growth after the war; members numbered 408 at mid-century. Figure 7-2 illustrates the dramatic growth in later years.

By 1954 membership had grown to 908; by 1964 to 1615, by 1974 to 2262, and by 1984 to more than 4000 members! At the Annual Meeting in 1983, 177 new members were elected, more than one and one-half times the number of charter members. By 1983 there were members of ARA in every state of the nation.

It is of interest that at the time of its formation, ARA encouraged lay membership and by 1939 had elected 83 lay members. With the formation of the Arthritis and Rheumatism Foundation, lay men and women interested in arthritis had a place for their activities in that organization and no longer became members of ARA. However, besides the active members, the ARA membership includes *emeritus* members, which totaled 142 in 1983. This low number of emeritus members reflects the relative youth of members when elected. A total of 110 persons recognized for their preeminence in the study or control of rheumatic diseases have been elected to *honorary* membership. All except seven of the honorary members are from foreign countries; only two are laymen, Mr. Edward Dunlop,

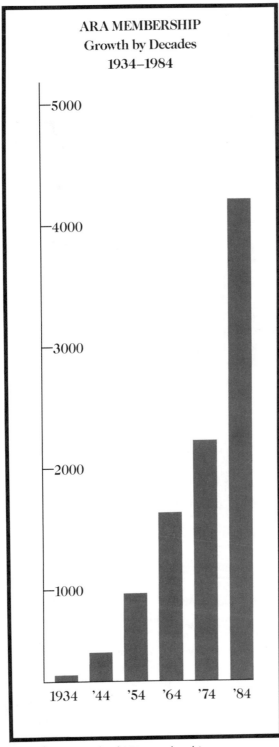

ARA MEMBERSHIP
Growth by Decades
1934–1984

5000

4000

3000

2000

1000

1934 '44 '54 '64 '74 '84

Figure 7-2. Growth of ARA membership.

who was President of the Canadian Arthritis and Rheumatism Society and Mr. Floyd B. Odlum, first Chairman of the Arthritis Foundation.

The rapid growth in membership of ARA is another impressive indication of the progress of American rheumatology.

EDUCATIONAL PUBLICATIONS

Primer. As mentioned in Chapter 3, the Metropolitan Life Insurance Company prepared and distributed a pamphlet titled "Rheumatic Diseases" in 1927. A booklet called "What Is Rheumatism?" issued by Metropolitan Life in 1930 included the statement, "Prepared in cooperation with the American Committee for the Control of Rheumatism." These two publications were the first of their kind on arthritis and rheumatism printed in the United States.

The first publication actually called a *Primer* was a small booklet entitled *Rheumatism Primer on Chronic Arthritis; Preliminary Printing*. It was prepared and privately published in 1932 "for the Medical Profession by a Sub-Committee of the American Committee for the Control of Rheumatism." Three thousand copies were printed and distributed. A note attached to a copy of this *Primer*, in Dr. Russell Haden's handwriting, reads, "This was prepared by the Committee and published with the aid of funds given to the Committee. Many of us had a hand in this. I believe I was the final Editor" (140).

The next version was a *Primer on Rheumatism, Chronic Arthritis* published in 1934 in the *Journal of the American Medical Association* (JAMA). This publication was the first edition of the *Primer* sponsored by the American Rheumatism Association (2). Dr. Edward Jordan, Associate Editor of *JAMA*, was the Editor. Reprints were made in a pocket-sized booklet. This first ARA *Primer* contained brief descriptions of the pathologic and clinical characteristics and basic treatment of the major forms of arthritis, aimed at assisting the practicing physician in diagnosis and patient care.

The *Primer* has undergone several revisions, each prepared by a committee of the ARA, with the Chairman acting as Editor-in-Chief (Table 7-1). The Editorial Committee for the 1983 (eighth) *Primer* had the assistance of a distinguished panel of 12 foreign authorities to review particular sections. This edition also contains contributions from 15 foreign rheumatologists.

The primary purpose of the *Primer* has always been to provide thorough but concise descriptions of the rheumatic diseases with emphasis on clinical manifestations, pathogenesis, diagnosis, and management. The *Primer* is widely used in the United States and abroad in teaching programs. It is distributed to members of ARA and AHPA and to medical schools and hospitals for students and house officers.

As knowledge of the rheumatic diseases grew, the *Primer* became larger and larger until the eighth (latest) edition contained 238 pages. In the 206 pages of text were 164 illustrations, 46 tables, and 11 pages of appendices. All of the *Primers* were published by JAMA until the eighth, which was issued by the Arthritis Foundation as a separate textbook. Recent editions of the *Primer* have become quite comprehensive elementary textbooks for arthritis and allied diseases. More than 250,000 copies of the seventh edition were distributed to physicians, medical students, and even many concerned patients.

The Rheumatism Reviews. At its 1932 meeting, the American Committee for the Study and Control of Rheumatism decided to make a comprehensive review of the English language articles on arthritis and rheumatism. The Committee appointed Dr. Philip Hench Chairman of a Review Subcommittee for this project. He was assigned to choose the other members of the Committee. The task was started promptly and the first *Review* was published in 1935 in the *Annals of Internal Medicine* (64). It was immediately recognized as a valuable educational publication, especially for the investigator and the clinical rheumatologist. The Rheumatism Review Committee was made a standing committee of the ARA, and plans were set to bring the literature review up to date at one- or two-year intervals. The *Reviews* continued to be published up to 1983. The last, the *Twenty-fifth*

Table 7-1. Growth of the *Primer on the Rheumatic Diseases, 1932–1983*

ARA Edition	Year Published	Where Published	Editor, Chairman of Editorial Committee	Pages of Text
	1932	Private	Russell Haden, MD	
1st	1934	JAMA	Edward Jordan, MD	
2nd	1942	JAMA	Edward Jordan, MD	16
3rd	1949	JAMA	Currier McEwen, MD	23
4th	1953	JAMA	Charles Ragan, MD	29
5th	1959	JAMA	Darrell C. Crain, MD	39
6th	1964	JAMA	John L. Decker, MD	71
7th	1973	JAMA	Gerald Rodnan, MD	154
8th	1983	Arthritis Foundation	Gerald Rodnan, MD and H. Ralph Schumacher, MD	206

Rheumatism Review, covered the literature of 1979–1980 and appeared in February, 1983 (90).

The format of the *Reviews* continued essentially the same from the first issue. The journal literature relating to each type of rheumatic disease is concisely summarized with editorial comments and criticisms liberally sprinkled in the text but always indicated as such. Each article reviewed is listed in the bibliography, which is a valuable part of each *Review*.

It is of interest that early editions contained a section reviewing the progress of the campaign against rheumatism; this review included the major activities of the ARA. The first 16 editions were published in the *Annals of Internal Medicine*; subsequent issues were printed as supplements or special issues of *Arthritis and Rheumatism*, except for the twentieth, which was published separately.

The *Rheumatism Reviews* stand as a tribute to Dr. Hench, whose inspiration and indefatigable energy accounted for their success. Dr. Hench served as Chairman of the Rheumatism Review Subcommittee and Editor-in-Chief through the ninth edition (1948), when he resigned. Succeeding him as Editor of the *Reviews* were: Dr. William D. Robinson through the eleventh issue (1956), Dr. Charley J. Smyth through the sixteenth (1964), Dr. Charles Christian through the nineteenth (1970), Dr. William M. Mikkelsen through the twenty-fourth (1981), and Dr. Thomas A. Medsger, the twenty-fifth (1983). All of Dr. Hench's successors carried on the high standard he set, maintaining the excellent tradition of the *Reviews*.

Arthritis and Rheumatism. The desire for an American rheumatism journal was slow to materialize. It was not until 14 years after formation of the American Rheumatism Association that serious consideration of an official ARA journal developed. This delay was in sharp contrast to the rapid development of arthritis and rheumatism journals in Europe during the 1930s and 1940s. The first of these journals was *Acta Rheumatologica*, which was started by Professor van Breemen in 1929. In 1934 the French *Revue du Rhumatisme* appeared; in 1936 and 1937 two rheumatism journals were started in Argentina; in 1938, one in Germany and two in Great Britain. In 1939 the *Annals of the Rheumatic Diseases* was introduced by the British Medical Association. Beginning in 1945, national rheumatism journals sprang up in Spain, Belgium, France, Italy, Yugoslavia, and Sweden.

Why was interest in a journal so slow to develop in the United States? There were several logical reasons. In the early days of the ARA, the principle was held that articles on arthritis and rheumatism should be published in conventional medical journals so they would be more widely read and spawn broader interest in rheumatism. Further, the success of the *Rheumatism Reviews* dampened interest in an American journal. Internationally acclaimed as important contributions to the advancement of knowledge in arthritis and rheumatism, the *Reviews* were considered, in a way, to take the place of a national journal. Also, in those days only a small number of good articles were submitted for publication internationally. Many ARA members believed that it would be wiser to support a single, strong English language journal, namely the *Annals of Rheumatic Diseases*, than to start a competing journal.

The first outspoken voice for an American rheumatism journal was that of Dr. Robert Stecher. In his presidential address to ARA in 1948, he made an earnest plea for the establishment of an official journal for the Association. "The time has come," he said, "when this Association must establish a journal of its own. Business of the organization is complex, important decisions must be made and an adequate medium of communication to the membership is essential" (140). But obstacles were in the way. The Editor of the British *Annals of Rheumatic Diseases* had expressed hope that this journal might be adopted as the official journal of the ARA. Early in the 1940s, the editorial board of the *Annals* had been enlarged to include ARA members as Associate Editors. Dr. Loring Swaim was the first appointed, soon followed by Dr. Philip Hench, and later by Drs. Edward Boland and Walter Bauer.

As interest in a completely American journal grew, the British, quite naturally, were reluctant to lose American editorial and reader support. Also, a small but influential group of pioneer members of ARA, including some past presidents, opposed the establishment of an ARA journal, fearing it would not be successful, doubting the existence of sufficient editorial talent within the membership, and deploring the competition to the *Annals* that would result from an American journal. But the ARA Executive Committee persisted in exploring the proposition further, and in November 1953, Dr. Joseph Hollander was appointed Chairman of the Committee on the Desirability and Feasibility of an American Journal on Arthritis and Rheumatism. This Committee studied all aspects of the matter, and Dr. Hollander gave a comprehensive report at the Executive Committee meeting in June 1954, stating that the Committee considered it feasible to start an ARA journal and so recommended. The Executive Committee, however, wanted further study before taking action. A poll of the ARA membership taken in 1955 showed that a majority of the members favored an official journal. However, the Executive Committee and membership of ARA did not vote for publication of a journal until 1957.

A Publication Committee for the journal, with Dr. Richard Freyberg as Chairman, was appointed and empowered to select an Editor-in-Chief and to contract for publication of the Journal. Dr. William S. Clark was appointed Editor. Dr. Clark had been strongly in favor of a journal; he was very concerned that it be successful and of the highest quality. He formed a strong editorial board. All worked diligently with Dr. Clark, who was inspirational, and the journal was carefully and meticulously planned. It was named *Arthritis and Rheumatism*, Official Journal of the American Rheumatism Association (A&R).

The first issue was published February 1958 (Figure 7-3). In his editorial in that volume, Dr. Clark foresaw that the new journal would "almost certainly become a highly significant medium for the exchange of scientific information among those concerned with the cause and cure of rheumatism" (24). Dr. Stecher, the journal's early advocate, predicted "a bright future for *Arthritis and Rheumatism*" (140).

Dr. Clark continued as Editor of *Arthritis and Rheumatism* until he resigned in 1965 to become President of the Arthritis Foundation. He was succeeded by Dr. Daniel J. McCarty until 1970; Dr. Charles L. Christian, 1970–75; Dr. J. Claude Bennett, 1975–80; Dr. Nathan J. Zvaifler, 1980–85.

Although Dr. McCarty reports having had problems finding enough worthwhile articles to fill 96 pages bimonthly, by the time of Dr. Bennett's editorship, sufficient material was available to increase the number of issues from six to 12 a year.

Examination of the contents over the years reveals a trend away from the clinical presentations and case reports of earlier volumes toward more scientific and research-oriented articles, especially after the mid-1970s. The advent of the multipurpose arthritis centers in 1977 led to more articles on the psychologic, sociologic, and economic aspects

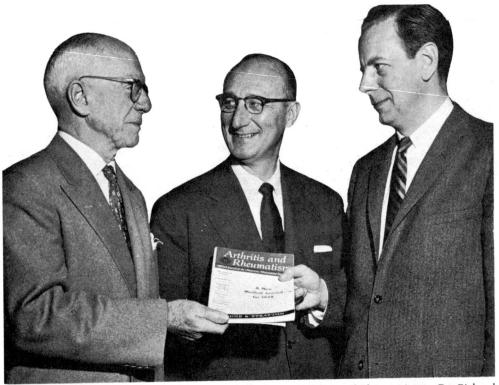

Figure 7-3. Dr. Russell Cecil (left) presenting first copy of *Arthritis and Rheumatism* to Dr. Richard Freyberg, Chairman of the Publication Committee (center) and Dr. William Clark, Editor (right).

of arthritis, often written by both physicians and allied health professionals. The waxing and waning of the theories about viruses in the etiology of rheumatic diseases, the romance with cortisone, the fascination with various forms of DNA, the intensified interest in lupus as the model for immunologic diseases, the scramble to find new HLA-disease associations, and the popularity of various mouse models can all be traced in the pages of *Arthritis and Rheumatism*. Even the journal's advertising reflects changes in the field of rheumatology. The tranquilizers and painkillers touted in early issues were later replaced by increasingly sophisticated ads for the newer nonsteroidal antiinflammatory drugs. Interestingly, rheumatologists have always shown appreciation for the broadest application of their specialty by publishing papers on the art, history, and poetry ("Arthritis is a Mean Disease" by Stephen Vincent Benet appeared in an early volume) of the rheumatic diseases, even including articles about arthritis on stamps.

Circulation grew to 7,890 by 1983, including 1,840 foreign subscriptions. The "die-hards" who for so long had opposed the journal's establishment became its staunch supporters.

Credit for sparking interest in an American journal for arthritis surely belongs to Dr. Stecher for persistently pursuing the project until its establishment; to Dr. Hollander and his committee for their optimism and careful investigation; and to Dr. Clark and his successors along with their editorial boards for the continued excellence of A&R. The American Rheumatism Association can well be proud of its official journal, *Arthritis and Rheumatism*, which has been internationally acclaimed for its high standards as a specialty journal for rheumatology.

Other Educational Projects. Several important educational projects that have not been an integral part of the ARA educational program have drawn heavily on the talents of prominent members of the Association. Examples are:

Bulletin on the Rheumatic Diseases. This publication, so valuable to the primary care physician, has been published and distributed by the Foundation. From the beginning, its editors have been prominent leaders of ARA, and the majority of articles have been contributed, on request of the editor, by clinical investigators and educators who are members of the Association (see Chapter 8).

Proceedings of Conferences. The Arthritis Foundation has conducted 18 conferences on subjects of special interest in rheumatic diseases in which many ARA members have participated. Presented papers and discussions have been published in monograph form as conference proceedings, often as issues of A&R. Association members have edited most of the Proceedings. The Arthritis Foundation Conference Series through 1975 is listed in the *Proceedings of the Conference on Pseudogout and Pyrophosphate Metabolism* (86).

Slide Collections. An unusual educational project has been the assembling and distribution of slides together with a syllabus for teaching of the rheumatic diseases. The first collection of lantern slides, prepared under the direction of Drs. Currier McEwen and Leon Sokoloff in 1956, featured illustrations of pathology of rheumatic diseases. It proved so valuable, particularly for medical students and house officers, that the Visual Aids Subcommittee of the Education Committee of the ARA was created to enlarge the scope of the first collection by adding slides of clinical and roentgenographic features of the rheumatic diseases.

This subcommittee was later enlarged to 14 members, with Dr. E. Carwile LeRoy as Chairman. Dr. Michael Lockshin worked closely with professional photographers Lester and Sylvia Bergman of New York to ensure the high technical quality of the 35 mm transparencies. In the development of the Collection, 10,000 slides submitted by 105 physicians were reviewed and 240 selected for inclusion in the teaching set. The development costs, which amounted to slightly less than $10,000, were underwritten by the Foundation. After three years of preparation, the *Clinical Slide Collection on the Rheumatic Diseases* was completed in 1972 and offered to rheumatologists and other physicians concerned with rheumatic diseases. Each set of slides was accompanied by a syllabus written by Drs. William Beetham and Jack Zuckner, including a black and white photograph of each slide.

In 1976 the Audiovisual Aids Subcommittee of the ARA Education Committee, under the Chairmanship of Dr. Joseph D. Croft, Jr., brought the 1972 Slide Collection up to date. Developmental costs were again underwritten by the Foundation. After a review of approximately 2,000 new slides, 40 were selected to replace some of the clinical and radiographic topics of the first Collection and 93 were chosen as additions. Nearly half the new slides depicted diseases with rheumatic manifestations not included in the previous edition, thus reflecting the increased knowledge about diagnosis of rheumatic diseases. The *Revised Clinical Slide Collection on the Rheumatic Diseases* was designed by the Committee to encourage ongoing revisions and additions. In 1981 this Revised Collection was published by the Arthritis Foundation. The work of adding to and modifying the Collection continued under the chairmanship of Dr. Sidney R. Block.

MERGER OF ARA AND THE ARTHRITIS AND RHEUMATISM FOUNDATION

As early as 1950, only two years after the formation of the Arthritis and Rheumatism Foundation, the idea of amalgamation of ARA with the Foundation was introduced in the ARA Executive Committee. Some difficulties in cooperation and coordination of activities of two separate organizations were surfacing. These problems arose chiefly within the Executive Committee and some of the subcommittees of the ARA. Because the ARA was required to provide members for the Medical and Scientific Committee of the Foundation and some of the Board of Directors, many ARA Executive Committee members found themselves serving on overlapping or completely duplicated committees. This entailed considerable time and effort by those persons sitting on both committees. Duplication also existed at the local level between the affiliated rheumatism societies and the Foundation chapters. Then, too, some leaders of the ARA wanted a greater voice in the Foundation's public relations efforts involving medical activities, clinic standards, and other professional activities. ARA members felt that closer coordination of the medical and scientific programs was needed.

So within the ARA, strong sentiment arose that consolidation of the ARA and the Foundation would obviate overlap and duplication of labor and significantly reduce the other problems existing between the two organizations. On the other hand, many of the older members and leaders of the ARA opposed amalgamation, fearing it would weaken the professional organization (ARA) of which they were so proud. This disagreement led to the appointment of an ARA Committee on Interrelationship of ARA and ARF to study the question further. The Foundation initially opposed the idea of merger. This question became a problem without solution. During the next three years, the pro-merger sentiment waned and the ad hoc Integration Committee was dissolved in 1955. The merger issue remained dormant for the next five years; both organizations prospered in their own ways.

In 1960 merger again became an important issue. ARA members underlined the need to eliminate duplication of efforts and emphasized the stronger leadership that would result from one integrated body. After all these years, the ARA and the Foundation had clearly become interdependent. Each realized it must look to the other for support and leadership. To act in unison, merger almost suggested itself. Both organizations looked for a suitable way to accomplish this unification.

After five years of study, it was proposed that the ARA merge into the Foundation and become a professional section of the Foundation but retain its name and independent internal organization. The bulk of the assets of the ARA were to be put in trust by the Foundation for five years so that if consolidation failed to satisfy the ARA, the merger could be dissolved and the Association could again become independent. This proposal was accepted by a vote of the ARA members at its annual meeting in 1965, and the Amalgamation and Trust Agreement was signed on June 30, 1965. On June 30, 1970 the remaining assets in trust were turned over to the Foundation, and the ARA conducted all its activities as the *American Rheumatism Association Section of the Arthritis Foundation*. The Foundation maintained the Delaware ARA Corporation as a shell organization to protect the name American Rheumatism Association from use by any other organization (see Chapter 8).

ESTABLISHMENT OF A SUBSPECIALTY BOARD
FOR RHEUMATOLOGY

In the early 1960s many ARA members expressed a desire for the establishment of a board of rheumatology for certification of physicians specializing in rheumatic diseases. This idea was discussed in several ARA Executive Committee meetings, but the proposal received little support until 1965, when an ARA Rheumatology Subspecialty Committee was appointed to study the matter. Dr. Joseph Hollander was appointed Chairman. Also on this committee was Dr. William Robinson, who was then on the American Board of Internal Medicine (ABIM). Dr. Robinson held strong views on recognizing rheumatology as a specialty. His philosophy was expressed emphatically in a paper titled "Rheumatology as a Subspecialty of Internal Medicine" (122), which he presented at the Arthritis Foundation sponsored *Third Conference on Education in Rheumatic Diseases* in September 1967. In this paper Dr. Robinson stated, "It should be emphasized that there is a very meaningful interrelationship between internal medicine and the field of rheumatic diseases," that "rheumatology *is* internal medicine," and that "too sharp a separation of rheumatology from the broader field of internal medicine would be a real loss both to the field of rheumatic diseases and to the field of internal medicine." He continued, "We quite clearly should not become so preoccupied with the status of rheumatology as a subspecialty that we lose sight of or weaken our efforts in improving the ability and resources of every physician who cares for the arthritic patient."

In concluding his discussion Dr. Robinson stated, "I would urge that the decision with respect to a subspecialty board of rheumatology be made on the basis of professional responsibility. If we can identify a body of knowledge and experience, beyond that needed in the broad field of internal medicine, which constitutes rheumatology, and are satisfied that there is a need for setting a standard by which people having such skills and experience can be recognized, then we clearly have a responsibility for the development of such a subspecialty board. The acid test should be whether such a development will really improve the care of patients with rheumatic diseases. And, finally, we should make this decision as members of a profession sufficiently responsive to the needs of society so that we continue to deserve the privilege of determining our own professional destinies."

The ARA ad hoc committee pondered Dr. Robinson's advice and studied all aspects of the matter for several years. Several conferences were held with the American Board of Internal Medicine. The Chairman reported to the ARA Executive Committee that the ad hoc committee could not come to a consensus regarding the desirability of a subspecialty board in rheumatology at that time and presented the pros and cons the committee had uncovered. The matter was debated in the Executive Committee through the following years, but no decision was made. Sometimes the debate was very lively!

The debate continued in ARA Executive Committee meetings with sentiment becoming increasingly favorable. In 1970 the ARA demonstrated an active interest in the development of rheumatology as a subspecialty of internal medicine and negotiated with the ABIM for the establishment of a subspecialty board. At its annual meeting in 1970, ARA voted in favor of a subspecialty board of rheumatology within the ABIM. In April 1971 the ABIM announced in the Medical News section of the *Annals of Internal Medicine* that a Subspecialty Board of Rheumatology had been established. Examinations for certification would be given at two-year intervals, the first in the fall of 1972. To qualify to take the

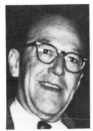
Edward F. Hartung
1960-61

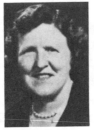
Marian W. Ropes
1963-64

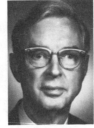
Howard F. Polley
1964-65

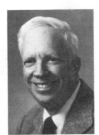
Donald F. Hill
1966-67

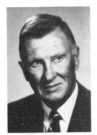
Evan Calkins
1967-68

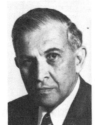
Edward E. Fischel
1968-69

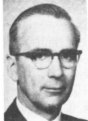
John H. Vaughn
1970-71

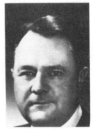
J. Sidney Stillman
1971-72

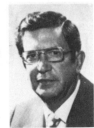
Thomas E. Weiss
1973-74

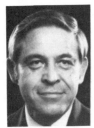
Giles G. Bole, Jr.
1980-81

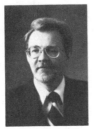
J. Claude Bennett
1981-82

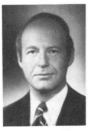
Gerald Weissmann
1982-83

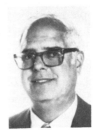
James R. Klinenberg
1983-84

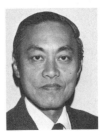
Eng M. Tan
1984-85

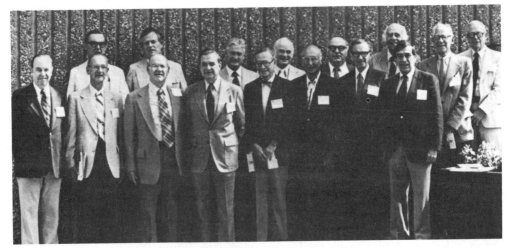
Past Presidents Attending Annual Session—Atlanta, 1980

Figure 7-4. ARA Presidents, 1959-1985. Group photo, back row, from left: John L. Decker, 1972–73, Charles L. Christian, 1976–77, Emmerson Ward, 1969–70, Daniel J. McCarty, 1979–80, Gerald P. Rodnan, 1975–76, Ephraim P. Engleman, 1962–63, Currier McEwen, 1952–53, Charley J. Smyth, 1959–60. Front row, from left: Carl M. Pearson, 1977–78, William D. Robinson, 1956–57, Joseph L. Hollander, 1961–62, Edward D. Boland, 1954–55, Alan S. Cohen, 1978–79, Richard H. Freyberg, 1948–49, Morris Ziff, 1965–66, Lawrence E. Shulman, 1974–75.

examination, the applicant had to be a diplomate of the ABIM and have had at least two years of subspecialty training.

Intensive review courses in rheumatic diseases were established by ARA to assist applicants in preparing for the Subspecialty Boards. These courses were given in the years the Subspecialty Board examinations were held.

Two hundred and one physicians took the first examination given in 1972; 154 passed to become the first board-certified specialists in rheumatology. By 1982 a total of 1,517 physicians had been certified by the Subspecialty Board of Rheumatology.

SPECIAL ARA PROJECTS

Practically all of the work of the Association, including special projects and publications, is accomplished through committees. In the 1982–83 *ARA–AHPA Membership Directory* are listed 11 standing committees established by ARA rules of procedure to conduct the more routine continuing work of the Association. The special projects are developed through ad hoc committees appointed by the President. In 1982–83 there were six such committees covering a wide range of activities. In recent years five ARA Councils were established to aid the work of clinicians and investigators especially interested in subdivisions of the broad field of rheumatology. All committees and councils are aided in the conduct of their business by a competent staff in the office of the Professional Societies Department of the Arthritis Foundation: Ms. Lynn Bonfiglio, Executive Secretary, who has been in this office since 1970, and her administrative staff Ms. Angel Fortenberry and Mr. Ronald F. Olejko.

Classification of Rheumatic Diseases. The lack of a standard rheumatologic nomenclature in the early 1900s was mentioned in Chapter 1. It is difficult for a physician of today to appreciate the confusion in terminology that existed before 1941. A striking example was the lack of clear distinction between degenerative and rheumatoid arthritis. In spite of the scholarly study of Nichols and Richardson in 1909, which established the pathologic differences between the two (98), confusion persisted. Twenty-six years later, in 1935, the twelfth edition of the standard medical text of the day, Osler's *The Principles and Practice of Medicine*, revised by Thomas McCrae, included both diseases under the heading arthritis deformans.

Although the term rheumatoid arthritis had been in rather general use in England since its introduction by Garrod in 1858, in the United States the disease was usually called chronic infectious arthritis because of the prevailing view that it was caused by focal infections. Other terms used were atrophic arthritis, especially by roentgenologists and orthopedists, and proliferative arthritis, the name adopted by Nichols and Richardson.

In 1940 a committee of the New York Rheumatism Association proposed a classification of rheumatic diseases (66), a proposal that spurred the American Rheumatism Association to undertake the development of a classification on a national scope. A committee was appointed consisting of Drs. Russell Cecil, Martin Dawson, Paul Holbrook, Currier McEwen, and Walter Bauer, with Bauer as chairman.

All the members were fully aware of the differences between degenerative arthritis and the basically inflammatory types. The committee readily chose the term rheumatoid arthritis. No one on the committee dissented from the view that articular involvement in patients with psoriasis or ulcerative colitis was merely rheumatoid arthritis that, for some reason, tended to occur in association with those diseases. Everyone also agreed on the separation of degenerative spondylitis from the spondylitis of Marie-Strümpell disease.

Table 7-2. Provisional classification adopted by ARA in 1941

1. Specific infectious arthritis (organism known)
2. Arthritis of rheumatic fever
3. Rheumatoid arthritis (synonyms: atrophic, proliferative and chronic nonspecific infectious arthritis, Still's disease, Marie-Strümpell spondylitis)
4. Osteoarthritis (synonyms: degenerative joint disease, hypertrophic, senescent arthritis)
5. Arthritis of immediate traumatic origin
6. Arthritis of gout
7. Arthritis of neuropathic origin (Charcot's joint)
8. Neoplasms of joints
9. Miscellaneous forms (or arthritis associated with other diseases)

There was, however, sharp disagreement about the nature of the latter, with Drs. Cecil and McEwen believing Marie-Strümpell spondylitis to be a distinct disease and the others considering it merely rheumatoid arthritis of the spine.

At the second meeting of the committee, Dr. Bauer reported some then-unpublished observations by Dr. Granville Bennett, the pathologist working with his group at Harvard. Dr. Bennett's studies showed that the histologic features of the lesions in the apophyseal joints in Marie-Strümpell spondylitis were like those in the synovial membrane of the peripheral joints in rheumatoid arthritis. The naivete of the knowledge of pathology at the time is well illustrated by the fact that such histologic similarities were accepted as indicating similar etiology. Drs. Cecil and McEwen, although reluctantly, agreed to adoption of the term rheumatoid spondylitis, a mistake that remained uncorrected for 23 years.

Imperfect as this classification adopted in 1941 was (65), it served an extremely important role in finally providing a common group of terms that quickly came into general use. Furthermore, the questions raised at the meetings of the committee stimulated intensive exploration of similarities and differences between what had, by then, been called the variants of rheumatoid arthritis. Later the evidence became convincing that ankylosing spondylitis, psoriatic arthritis, Reiter's syndrome, and the arthritis accompanying ulcerative colitis and regional enteritis were separate entities distinct from rheumatoid arthritis (35, 88). As a result, a new committee on nomenclature and classification was appointed by the ARA to prepare a revised classification, which was adopted in 1964 (14). With passing years, newly recognized rheumatic diseases were added to the already formidable array of diseases affecting the joints, and the classification of 1964 was brought up to date as new information dictated (127). Meanwhile, the new classification, like its very imperfect predecessor of 1941, provided a common terminology for all to use.

The striking developments in classification and recognition of additional rheumatic diseases are well illustrated by comparing the first classification adopted by the ARA in 1941, Table 7-2, with that published in the *Primer on the Rheumatic Diseases* (eighth edition) in 1983 (127), Table 7-3.

Diagnostic Criteria. Distinct from these efforts to formulate general classifications were efforts sponsored by the ARA and Arthritis Foundation to establish criteria for various individual diseases. The first of these (142) was concerned with criteria for evaluating a patient's stage of articular damage and functional capacity as guides in prescribing a rational program of treatment. Subsequently a series of committees undertook the development of diagnostic criteria.

The first set of criteria, on rheumatoid arthritis (128, 129), was a model for those that followed and serves well to illustrate the difficulties involved and the approach taken

I. Diffuse connective tissue diseases
  A. Rheumatoid arthritis
  B. Juvenile arthritis
    1. Systemic onset
    2. Polyarticular onset
    3. Oligarticular onset
  C. Systemic lupus erythematosus
  D. Progressive systemic sclerosis
  E. Polymyositis/dermatomyositis
  F. Necrotizing vasculitis and other vasculopathies
    1. Polyarteritis nodosa group (includes hepatitis B associated arteritis and Churg-Strauss allergic granulomatosis)
    2. Hypersensitivity vasculitis (includes Schönlein-Henoch purpura and others)
    3. Wegener's granulomatosis
    4. Giant cell arteritis
      a. Temporal arteritis
      b. Takayasu's arteritis
    5. Mucocutaneous lymph node syndrome (Kawasaki's disease)
    6. Behcet's disease
  G. Sjogren's syndrome
  H. Overlap syndromes (includes mixed connective tissue disease)
  I. Others (includes polymyalgia rheumatica, panniculitis (Weber-Christian disease), erythema nodosum, relapsing polychondritis, and others)
II. Arthritis associated with spondylitis
  A. Ankylosing spondylitis
  B. Reiter's syndrome
  C. Psoriatic arthritis
  D. Arthritis associated with chronic inflammatory bowel disease
III. Degenerative joint disease (osteoarthritis, osteoarthrosis)
  A. Primary (includes erosive osteoarthritis)
  B. Secondary
IV. Arthritis, tenosynovitis, and bursitis associated with infectious agents
  A. Direct
    1. Bacterial
      a. Gram-positive cocci (staphylococcus and others)
      b. Gram-negative cocci (gonococcus and others)
      c. Gram-positive rods
      d. Mycobacteria
      e. Treponemes
      f. Others
    2. Viral
    3. Fungal
    4. Parasitic
    5. Unknown, suspected (Whipple's disease)
  B. Indirect (reactive)
    1. Bacterial (includes acute rheumatic fever, intestinal bypass, postdysenteric—shigella, yersinia, and others)
    2. Viral (hepatitis B)
V. Metabolic and endocrine diseases associated with rheumatic states
  A. Crystal-induced conditions
    1. Monosodium urate (gout)
    2. Calcium pyrophosphate dihydrate (pseudogout, chondrocalcinosis)
    3. Hydroxyapatite

Table 7-3 continued

B. Biochemical abnormalities
  1. Amyloidosis
  2. Vitamin C deficiency (scurvy)
  3. Specific enzyme deficiency states (includes Fabry's, Farber's, alkaptonuria, Lesch-Nyhan, and others)
  4. Hyperlipidemias (types II, IIa, IV)
  5. Mucopolysaccharides
  6. Hemoglobinopathies (SS disease and others)
  7. True connective tissue disorders (Ehlers-Danlos, Marfan's, pseudoxanthoma elasticum, and others)
  8. Others
C. Endocrine diseases
  1. Diabetes mellitus
  2. Acromegaly
  3. Hyperparathyroidism
  4. Thyroid disease (hyperthyroidism, hypothyroidism)
D. Immunodeficiency diseases
E. Other hereditary disorders
  1. Arthrogryposis multiplex congenita
  2. Hypermobility syndromes
  3. Myositis ossificans progressiva
VI. Neoplasms
A. Primary (e.g. synovioma, synoviosarcoma)
B. Metastatic
VII. Neuropathic disorders
A. Charcot joints
B. Compression neuropathies
  1. Peripheral entrapment (carpal tunnel syndrome and others)
  2. Radiculopathy
  3. Spinal stenosis
C. Reflex sympathetic dystrophy
D. Others
VIII. Bone and cartilage disorders associated with articular manifestations
A. Osteoporosis
  1. Generalized
  2. Localized (regional)
B. Osteomalacia
C. Hypertrophic osteoarthropathy
D. Diffuse idiopathic skeletal hyperostosis (includes ankylosing vertebral hyperostosis—Forestier's disease)
E. Osteitis
  1. Generalized (osteitis deformans—Paget's disease of bone)
  2. Localized (osteitis condensans ilii; osteitis pubis)
F. Avascular necrosis
G. Osteochondritis (osteochondritis dissecans)
H. Congenital dysplasia of the hip
I. Slipped capital femoral epiphysis
J. Costochondritis (includes Tietze's syndrome)
K. Osteolysis and chondrolysis
IX. Nonarticular rheumatism
A. Myofascial pain syndromes
  1. Generalized (fibrositis, fibromyalgia)
  2. Regional
B. Low back pain and intervertebral disc disorders

Table 7-3 continued

   C. Tendinitis (tenosynovitis) and/or bursitis
      1. Subacromial/subdeltoid bursitis
      2. Bicipital tendinitis, tenosynovitis
      3. Olecranon bursitis
      4. Epicondylitis, medial or lateral humeral
      5. DeQuervain's tenosynovitis
      6. Adhesive capsulitis of the shoulder (frozen shoulder)
      7. Trigger finger
   D. Ganglion cysts
   E. Fasciitis
   F. Chronic ligament and muscle strain
   G. Vasomotor disorders
      1. Erythromelalgia
      2. Raynaud's disease or phenomenon
   H. Miscellaneous pain syndromes (includes weather sensitivity, psychogenic rheumatism)
X. Miscellaneous disorders
   A. Disorders frequently associated with arthritis
      1. Trauma (the result of direct trauma)
      2. Lyme arthritis
      3. Pancreatic disease
      4. Sarcoidosis
      5. Palindromic rheumatism
      6. Intermittent hydrarthrosis
      7. Villonodular synovitis
      8. Hemophilia
   B. Other conditions
      1. Internal derangement of joints (includes chondromalacia patella, loose bodies)
      2. Familial Mediterranean fever
      3. Eosinophilic fasciitis
      4. Chronic active hepatitis
      5. Other drug-induced rheumatic syndromes

From the Primer on the Rheumatic Diseases, ed. 8, Atlanta, Arthritis Foundation, 1983, pp 36–37.

to overcome them. Major problems were the various manifestations of the disease in different patients and the lack of a single clinical feature or laboratory test of complete diagnostic reliability. The committee charged with responsibility for these criteria proposed 11 individual features and assigned greater or lesser certainty of diagnosis depending on the number of these features shown by a given patient. Thus the presence of 7 or more warranted a diagnosis of classical rheumatoid arthritis, whereas the presence of 5, 3, or 2 justified the diagnosis of definite, probable, or possible rheumatoid arthritis, respectively.

    These criteria proved so valuable that they have been used throughout the world, and their success led to similar undertakings by subsequent committees. Criteria were published for the diagnosis of systemic lupus erythematosus in 1971 (27), revised in 1982 (149); juvenile rheumatoid arthritis in 1972 (16), revised in 1977 (17); acute gouty arthritis in 1977 (163); progressive systemic sclerosis in 1980 (preliminary) (84); and for establishing clinical remission of rheumatoid arthritis in 1981 (110). Other committees were appointed to prepare criteria for the diagnosis of osteoarthritis and the classification of vasculitis.

    Cooperative Clinic Studies of New Forms of Therapy. As clinical investigation progressed, new therapeutic agents were developed, and clinical trials were needed to establish their value and tolerance. Reports of early studies from different clinics were often conflicting; selection of patients differed, protocols of study varied, and often studies were too brief or lacked controls. It became apparent that to obtain reliable information regarding new forms of therapy, it would be necessary to have longer studies of a large number of patients, following standard protocol, with statistical analysis of results. These requirements could best be fulfilled if several rheumatism clinics combined their efforts in interinstitutional studies. Recognizing this need, the ARA established a Committee for Cooperating Clinics to make controlled evaluation of new medications and therapeutic agents of unproven value. Over the years the cooperating clinics have evaluated many medications. Results of these cooperative studies have been published, usually in *Arthritis and Rheumatism*. (See Chapter 11.)

Evaluation of Synovectomy. A special evaluation was made of synovectomy (the surgical removal of the diseased lining membrane of joints). This procedure was claimed by many orthopedists to be curative in rheumatoid arthritic joints so treated. Because synovectomy was being performed with increasing frequency and earlier in the course of disease, a careful assessment of its true value was urgently needed. A committee consisting of two orthopedic surgeons, Drs. Carroll Larson and Louis Paradies; a physiatrist, Dr. Edwin Smith; a statistician, Dr. Donald Mainland; and two rheumatologists, Drs. Evan Calkins and Currier McEwen, the latter as chairman, prepared the protocol for a controlled, prospective, multicenter evaluation. The project was subsequently sponsored by the AF with financial support from the AF and NIAMD, the Ralph B. Rogers Foundation, and the Maine Chapter of the AF (see Chapter 11).

Uniform Database for Rheumatic Diseases. In September 1973 the ARA sponsored a Database Workshop, which resulted in the first version of "A Standard Database for Rheumatic Diseases" (67). A revision, titled "A Uniform Database for Rheumatic Diseases" (68), was published after the second Database Workshop held in September 1975. At a third Workshop in September 1978, the Database underwent intense review and revision (69). This database was the beginning of the ARA Medical Information System (ARAMIS) project. An important need identified at this workshop was the requirement for uniform definitions of many of the terms used in rheumatology. To meet this need, the ARA Glossary Committee was appointed, with Dr. John Decker as Chairman. The product of this Committee was the *Dictionary of the Rheumatic Diseases* published in September 1982 (33).

8

Growth and Contributions of the Arthritis Foundation

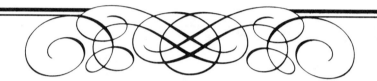

O N April 4, 1948, the Certificate of Incorporation of the Arthritis and Rheumatism Foundation (ARF) was filed in the State of New York and the predecessor of the current Arthritis Foundation (AF) was established. Mr. Floyd Odlum, the first Chairman of the Board of Directors, held this position for the next 22 years and ably led this rapidly developing organization through its early and often turbulent years into a nationwide network of chapters. Further details about the genesis and early developments of the Foundation are contained in Chapters 4 and 5. During most of these first two decades, the Foundation and its sponsoring body, the American Rheumatism Association, were separate self-governing organizations existing in symbiosis, i.e., they worked together in intimate and advantageous association. After 17 years of cohabitation in what may seem "an incestuous relationship" as it was called by Dr. Daniel McCarty (85), then President of the ARA, the ARA became amalgamated with the Arthritis and Rheumatism Foundation in 1965. That same year, the Arthritis and Rheumatism Foundation shortened its name to the Arthritis Foundation (AF).

When the Foundation began, the medical and scientific affairs were administered by Dr. Russell Cecil, a major figure in American medicine and rheumatology who served as the Consulting Medical Director for three years. He was followed by Dr. Gideon K. de Forest, of the Yale University Medical School, who was the first full-time Medical Director for the Foundation and served for the next five years.

THE FIRST 10 YEARS (1948–1958)

During the first decade, the Arthritis and Rheumatism Foundation made remarkable progress toward its goals, namely, wider public awareness of the magnitude of the problems of arthritis, better treatment facilities for arthritis sufferers, increased knowledge of the rheumatic diseases by health care providers, and the support of research aimed at tracking down the causes of these crippling diseases.

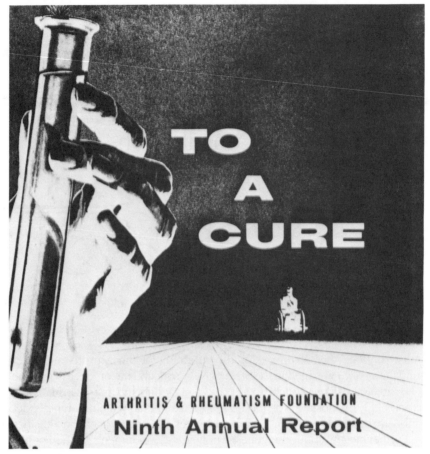

Figure 8-1. Cover of Arthritis and Rheumatism Foundation Annual Report, 1957.

Chapters Developed Nationwide. During the first 10 years, the number of chapters nationwide rapidly increased to 53, with services rendered to patients in 43 states and the District of Columbia. Support was provided to 200 arthritis treatment units, and during 1958 alone, 35 traveling clinics provided 77,000 physical therapy visits to homebound victims of arthritis. A study financed by the New York Chapter showed that an unexpectedly high percentage of patients disabled by arthritis could find employment through rehabilitation programs.

Support of Arthritis Research. As soon as the Foundation had been established, its lay and medical leaders recognized the need for training physicians and other scientists in this long-neglected field of medicine. A Research Fellowship Program was the first effort developed to meet this need and it was given high priority. During the first 10 years, $1,347,032 was contributed for its support (Figure 8-1). A 1976 review of the records of 34 of the fellows sponsored during the initial 10-year period revealed that 80% were still in rheumatology and 25 were in teaching and research institutions. Many leaders in arthritis research were among this group.

When the Foundation was young, only a few physicians were in the private practice of rheumatology so that in many areas people with arthritis had difficulty finding expert care. The local chapters of the Foundation recognized this problem and in 1958 gave $258,451 for 57 clinical fellowships for internists wishing to specialize in arthritis.

Development of Educational Programs. From the beginning, the Arthritis and Rheumatism Foundation placed major emphasis on the enormously important area of professional and lay education programs. Through newspapers, radio, television, and national magazines, the level of public knowledge of arthritis was raised. Handbooks for patients provided a valuable means of helping to explain the diseases. In this first decade, the number of training centers for physicians increased from eight to 32. In one year (1958), the chapters throughout the country contributed a total of $58,172 to these training centers for 32 clinical traineeships.

Bulletin on Rheumatic Diseases. This publication was created in 1950 by the New York Chapter of the Arthritis Foundation, with Dr. Joseph Bunim as editor. Its aim was to provide specialists and general physicians brief authoritative reviews of the current status of research and clinical practice in arthritis and related musculoskeletal disorders. In its 35 years, ARA members have served as editors of and contributors to the *Bulletin*. In 1984 the Editorial Board was expanded to include a family physician, an orthopedist, and a physical therapist. The *Bulletin* has been distributed without charge to interested health providers; in 1966 its circulation was 40,000 per issue and since then has grown to more than 45,000.

The immediate and continued success of these timely and practical reviews reflects the ability of its four editors: Dr. Joseph J. Bunim, the founder; Dr. Ronald W. Lamont-Havers, who served as interim editor for two years after Dr. Bunim's death; Dr. Gerald P. Rodnan, who held the editorship from 1966 to 1983; and Dr. Evelyn V. Hess, the current Editor. Under Dr. Rodnan, the publication grew in status and usefulness and achieved an unexcelled worldwide reputation for concise and accurate reporting by experts. Through this medium, the latest knowledge of the rheumatic diseases has been disseminated annually in 6 to 9 issues in 34 volumes. This AF sponsored publication has contributed much to the advancement of rheumatology as a growing specialty and is a tribute to the editors, the Editorial Board, and its contributing authors.

Postgraduate Seminars. Another avenue for reaching doctors and other professionals with the latest techniques in diagnosis and treatment has been through postgraduate seminars. In 1958 more than $100,000 was devoted to financing special seminars for physicians, nurses, and therapists. Such specialized courses sponsored over the years have resulted in a marked increase in interest in the rheumatic diseases.

NATIONAL FOUNDATION–MARCH OF DIMES (POLIO) ENTERS THE FIELD OF ARTHRITIS

In 1958 after Dr. Jonas Salk's discovery of an effective vaccine that almost eradicated polio, the National Foundation (NF) added arthritis to the list of diseases it would support. During the next six years, support was given to a number of universities for clinical study and for special treatment centers for children with rheumatic fever and other connective tissue diseases. In 1964 the National Foundation announced its plan to withdraw from the field of arthritis to concentrate its efforts on birth defects. This major development was accomplished through lengthy negotiations between Mr. Floyd Odlum and other officers of the Arthritis and Rheumatism Foundation and Mr. Basil O'Connor representing the National Foundation. At the same time Dr. William Clark, who had directed the rheumatic disease

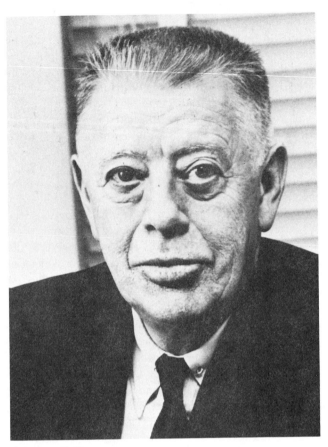

Figure 8-2. General George C. Kenney.

clinical centers for the NF, was named as successor to the first salaried full-time ARF President, General George Kenney (Figure 8-2). In accepting this position, Dr. Clark said, "The enormous menace arthritis presents to the health of America deserves the devoted attention of a single organization strong enough to cope with the nationwide effects of this affliction. We hope to enlist for our organization the interest and support of everyone, lay and professional, who wants to put an end to the misery of arthritis." When he took office in 1964, the Foundation became, as it remains today, the single voluntary organization with national responsibility for arthritis, including patient care, research, public and professional education, and fundraising.

FOUNDATION SHOWS STEADY GROWTH AND DEVELOPMENT

The Character of the AF Molded by Superior Lay Leadership. Since the Foundation came into existence, it has grown to be one of the leading voluntary health agencies in the United States. Today it is the only organization espousing the cause of more than 36 million people, including 250,000 children, afflicted with some type of arthritis or allied musculoskeletal disease. The activities of 71 chapters and divisions that span the nation from coast to coast are coordinated from the national office in Atlanta. This network involves approximately 400 salaried staff members and 400,000 volunteers. Each chapter

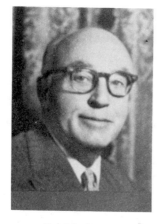

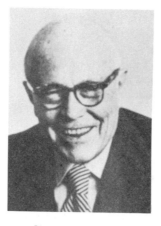

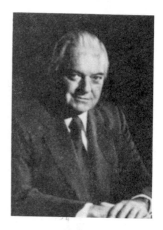

Floyd B. Odlum
1948–70

Charles B. Harding
1970–76

H M Poole, Jr.
1976–78

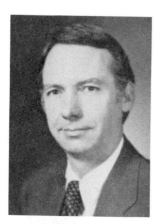

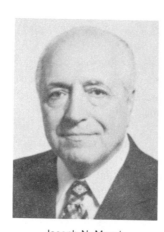

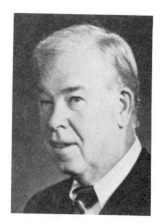

W. W. Satterfield
1978–80

Joseph N. Masci
1980–82

Edward J. Malone
1982–84

Figure 8-3. Chairmen of the Board of Directors of the Arthritis and Rheumatism Foundation, later Arthritis Foundation.

and division, depending upon its size, sends elected members as representatives to serve on the House of Delegates. From this group representing the chapters and from the officers and members of the Sections of the ARA and Arthritis Health Professions Association (AHPA) is chosen the Board of Trustees. In 1983 the Board consisted of 39 members: 11 physicians, four health professionals, and 24 lay volunteers. The Chairman of this board is elected by the House of Delegates. As of 1984, six outstanding business leaders had held this high position (Figure 8-3).

To a great extent, the early success and phenomenal growth of this health agency can be attributed to the first Chairman, Mr. Floyd Odlum of New York, himself a victim of rheumatoid arthritis. Through his unselfish devotion, his intellectual strength, and his extraordinary ability to select and attract others of exceptional talent and quality, he carefully molded the character of this nationwide movement.

His successor, Mr. Charles B. Harding, further shaped the destiny of this organization for the next six years (1970–1976). To him goes the credit of keeping unity within the organization through turbulent times. He succeeded in bringing together the widely scattered chapters, each with diverse grassroots activities, into a more effective organization. The highest Foundation award for volunteers is named in honor of Mr. Harding.

Through the administrative skills and competent leadership of these first two chairmen and those who followed (H M Poole, Jr., 1976–78; W. W. Satterfield, 1978–80; Joseph N. Masci, 1980–82; Edward J. Malone, 1982–84), the Foundation has shown steady growth and increasing stability. It has also obtained increasing financial support. Strong evidence that the American public has an awareness of the magnitude of the arthritis problem and confidence in the Arthritis Foundation and its leadership is indicated by the public support of more than $31 million in 1983. In addition, through its national and state government affairs committees, the Foundation has encouraged state and federal governments to provide greater financial support. In 1982 the Congress of the United States spent $62 million on arthritis programs, and several state legislatures have appropriated funds for arthritis.

Support of Medical Research and Training. In 1966, when the March of Dimes abandoned the field of arthritis, the Arthritis Foundation assumed financial responsibility for six arthritis research centers that had been established in 1958. During the next decade, the number of grants to medical and academic units increased and the title, Arthritis Clinical Research Center, became a mark of overall excellence for any arthritis program engaged in research, teaching, and patient care.

The flexibility of the funds granted to centers has allowed the centers to function when funding gaps occur, equipment must be replaced, or interesting new scientific directions require immediate investigation. Because the centers provide excellent teaching environments, many Foundation-supported fellows train in them (57).

In 1984, another type of center grant was established—the Biomedical Research Center Grant for centers of excellence in research. Currently, the Foundation supports 51 Arthritis Clinical Research Centers and two affiliated Arthritis Pediatric Centers in 28 states.

The Research Fellowship Program has remained the highest priority of the AF. Two additional fellowship programs, the Clinical Scholar and the Senior Fellowship Award (later Senior Investigator), were established in the 1960s. These five-year awards were given to a small number of individuals who had completed fellowship training and demonstrated both scientific independence and unusual ability and promise as clinical and basic investigators (41).

In 1983 these awards were replaced by the Arthritis Investigator Awards, designed to help scientists who had completed initial postdoctoral research training to become established researchers.

Postdoctoral fellowships, granted since 1951, provide for an initial period of training for physician and PhD scientists. In 1976, at a gathering of many former fellows to

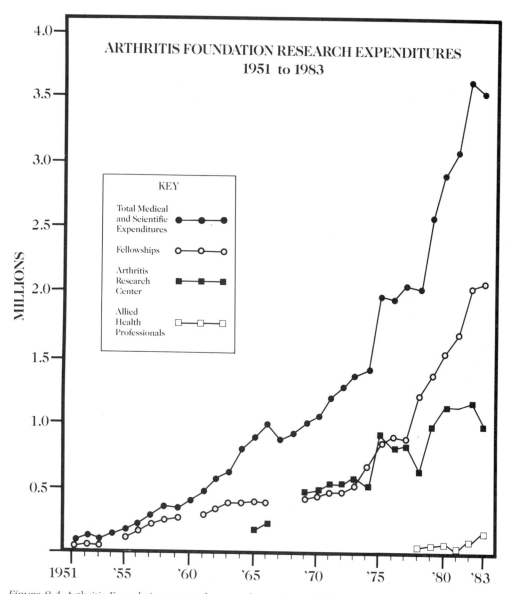

Figure 8-4. Arthritis Foundation research expenditures from 1951 to 1983.

celebrate the 25th anniversary of the AF fellowship program, it was announced that Baruch Blumberg had become the first former Foundation fellow to receive the Nobel Prize for Physiology and Medicine, for his work in identifying the Hepatitis B virus.

Expenditures for training of investigators in research and patient care have increased progressively since 1951 (Figure 8-4). By 1983 more than 600 physicians and scientists had received fellowships from the AF and hundreds of others had been trained through the Clinical Research Center program. About $33 million has been invested in these fellowships and grants. In 1982–83 there were 13 senior investigators, 7 investigators, 85 postdoctoral fellows, and 9 arthritis health professional fellows.

In 1977 an allied health professionals fellowship and grants program was established to train nonphysician investigators in health care research related to arthritis and to provide grants to investigators in these fields. By 1983 the traineeship program for allied health professionals had become focused on postdoctoral training of physical and occupational therapists, nurses, social workers, and other health professionals, and the grants program concentrated on the support of full-time investigators in these fields.

The Arthritis Foundation research program has evolved as well as expanded. The Arthritis Investigator Award was created in response to a study that demonstrated a great need for support in the crucial years immediately following completion of postdoctoral training. Recognition of the importance of research by allied health professionals more than 10 years ago resulted in the initiation of the grants program to train new investigators. In 1981 the Chapter Research Subcommittee, a peer review system for chapter-supported research, was established to help chapters avoid conflicts of interest in rating research projects and to ensure that the Foundation supports the highest quality research. Pediatric centers became eligible for center grants. In the 1970s representation by lay members on the research committee and its subcommittees was expanded.

These innovations indicate the Foundation's constant reexamination of the research program and its ability to respond to the needs of the scientific community.

Campaign Launched Against Arthritis Quackery. When the Arthritis and Rheumatism Foundation came into existence in 1948, the use of unproven remedies for the treatment of various types of arthritis represented a major expenditure by the American people. Although this unfortunate situation had existed for generations, during the middle to late 1950s the plethora of unproven claims of cures and quack remedies for arthritis was intensified by the publication of popular books on folk medicine cures and the establishment of clinics where inappropriate drug regimens were administered.

In response to this problem, the New York Chapter established a Committee on Arthritis Advertising in 1958, and Mrs. Ruth Walrad was employed as a research coordinator. A conference on "Misleading Advertising Regarding Arthritis Remedies," held in January 1959, was attended by members of the New York Chapter and by Dr. Ronald Lamont-Havers, Medical Director of the Arthritis and Rheumatism Foundation. By December of that year, a nationwide survey to obtain information on the extent of deceitful arthritis advertising and promotion of unproven products for the treatment of arthritis was completed, and the results were reported by the Foundation in May 1960. It was discovered that the quackery business in the United States was bigger in arthritis than in any other disease. The survey also revealed that charlatans and promoters of unproven remedies were cheating arthritis sufferers out of $250,000,000 annually.

"This report," recalls Dr. Lamont-Havers, "was an immediate success and brought the Foundation great acclaim from Federal regulating agencies, voluntary and professional organizations, and arthritis patients. A campaign of popular articles and presentations based on this report was begun" (76).

Shortly after the issuance of this report, Mr. Jerry Walsh, a young man with severe crippling arthritis but an undaunted spirit, joined the staff of the national office of the Foundation. Mr. Walsh made the misrepresentation campaign his own and lectured throughout the country making a striking impression. He effectively and forcefully championed the victims of arthritis and espoused their need to be protected from those who would exploit them. Shortly before his death in 1975, in recognition for his work, he

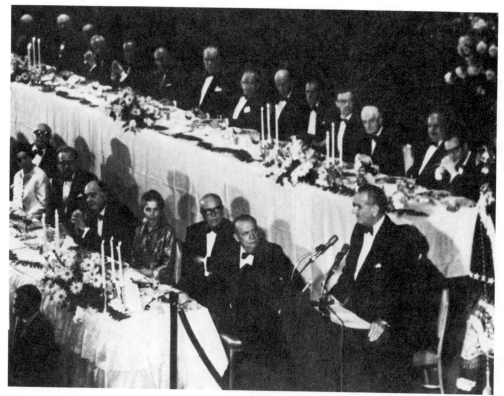

Figure 8-5. President Lyndon B. Johnson addressing the 20th anniversary dinner of the Arthritis Foundation.

was named the Handicapped American of the Year by the President's Committee on the Handicapped.

This program of the AF continues through its nationwide network of chapters using every channel of communication. Arthritis patients and their families are informed of the clever and sophisticated promotional methods of the modern day sales pitch for the "quick-cure" by the use of untested drugs and devices, irreputable clinics, and unestablished nutritional claims. Also, this program warns of the unreliability of personal testimonials favoring unproven remedies (copper bracelets, vaccines, acupuncture, herbs, vitamins, sea water, special diets, green-lipped mussel extract, and many more). It points out that although such evidence might sound convincing, it cannot be considered proof that the remedy works. Such testimonials are unreliable because of the "placebo effect" and the fact that the activity and the pain of the chronic forms of arthritis fluctuate so that the apparent beneficial effects may actually be due to spontaneous remissions or the natural course of these unpredictable illnesses. The campaign also emphasizes that scientifically designed and conducted trials of drugs and other remedies to measure safety and effectiveness are the only reliable proof of benefits.

A Celebration of 20 Years of Progress and Accomplishment. On May 20, 1968 in New York City, the President of the United States, Lyndon B. Johnson, said, "Surely no more vexing health problem can be named than the one that you battle, arthritis. . . Like

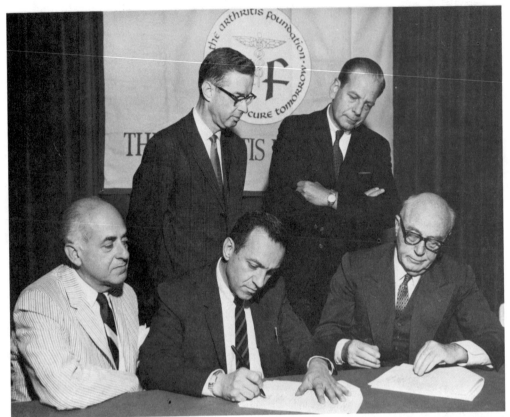

Figure 8-6. The ARA and the AF join forces in 1965. The merger agreement was signed by Mr. Floyd Odlum, Chairman of the Board of Directors of the AF (lower right) and Dr. Morris Ziff, President of the ARA. They are flanked by Drs. Ephraim P. Engleman (lower left) and Howard F. Polley (upper left) representing the officers of the ARA and Dr. William S. Clark, President of the AF (upper right).

most of our problems, it is within our power to solve it. If we have the will, we'll find the way." He was speaking at the 20th anniversary celebration dinner of the Arthritis Foundation (Figure 8-5). As the Foundation entered its third decade, great progress had already been accomplished, and the arthritis movement that had been started continues.

THE ARA AND AF JOIN FORCES

As both the ARA and the Foundation became increasingly aware that they were interdependent for support, leaders of both groups began to recognize the benefits of working in unison. An ad hoc ARA Committee on Interrelationship with ARF was appointed, with Dr. Ephraim P. Engleman Chairman, to explore ways to unify. Largely because he led the group with the skill of a true statesman, this committee after hours of study, stormy debate, and lengthy negotiations, submitted a plan acceptable to both parties.

On June 30, 1965, after five years of diligent effort, an amalgamation agreement was signed by Mr. Floyd Odlum, Chairman of the Board of Directors of AF, and Dr. Morris Ziff, President of ARA. That year the ARA became the professional wing of the AF (the ARA Section of the AF) (Figure 8-6).

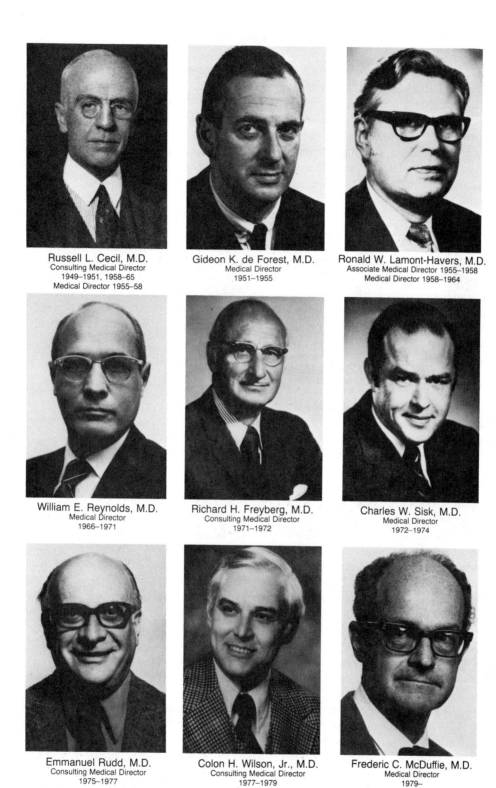

Russell L. Cecil, M.D.
Consulting Medical Director
1949–1951, 1958–65
Medical Director 1955–58

Gideon K. de Forest, M.D.
Medical Director
1951–1955

Ronald W. Lamont-Havers, M.D.
Associate Medical Director 1955–1958
Medical Director 1958–1964

William E. Reynolds, M.D.
Medical Director
1966–1971

Richard H. Freyberg, M.D.
Consulting Medical Director
1971–1972

Charles W. Sisk, M.D.
Medical Director
1972–1974

Emmanuel Rudd, M.D.
Consulting Medical Director
1975–1977

Colon H. Wilson, Jr., M.D.
Consulting Medical Director
1977–1979

Frederic C. McDuffie, M.D.
Medical Director
1979–

Figure 8-7. Medical directors and consulting medical directors of the Arthritis Foundation.

Medical Directors Play Key Role in Progress. One of the first steps taken by the Medical and Scientific Committee when the Arthritis and Rheumatism Foundation was newly established was to recommend to the Board of Directors the appointment of Dr. Russell Cecil as its Chief Medical Administrative Officer. This selection was exceedingly fortunate. He was an internationally recognized authority in medical education with outstanding research accomplishments in the rheumatic diseases. The wise counsel and guidance of this highly respected leader in American medicine from 1948 to 1951 set a high standard of excellence for the new voluntary health agency.

Since then, this office has been ably served by eight physicians either as full-time appointees or in a consulting role (Figure 8-7). The influence of this group of dedicated physicians upon research, training, patient care, and lay education in the rheumatic diseases has been remarkable. A partial list of their contributions includes: the progressive increase in the number of fellowships available, the excellence of the national and regional scientific meeting programs including poster sessions, teaching aids and slide collections, scientific publications, and pamphlets for patients on specific rheumatic diseases and aspects of treatment. Without the guidance and administrative help of the medical directors within the Arthritis Foundation, the useful programs and publications could not have been accomplished.

REORGANIZATION OF THE FOUNDATION IN 1976

For 11 years after the union of the ARA and AF in 1965, the medical and scientific affairs were regularly reviewed by a Foundation Medical Administrative Committee (MAC), which was composed of the Executive Committee of the ARA Section of the Foundation, nine regional representatives from the Arthritis Foundation chapters, one AHPA representative, and one lay representative from the AF board. With the rapid expansion of activities throughout the country and the appointment of Clifford M. Clarke as its President, the AF underwent a major reorganization in 1976. The aim was to increase efficiency and improve communications between the local and national staff and both the professional and lay volunteers.

The bylaws of the Foundation were changed to create two governing bodies, the House of Delegates and the Board of Trustees. The House of Delegates became the supreme governing body of the Foundation. Members were appointed or elected from the nationwide chapters on the basis of their contributions to the national budget. In addition, the presidents of the two professional sections (ARA and AHPA) were made officers of the Foundation. Delegates were also allotted later to the American Juvenile Arthritis Organization, and a certain number of positions were filled by professional and lay delegates elected at large. The House of Delegates meets once a year to act on the annual budget and to establish policy. During the year, the smaller Board of Trustees manages the business and affairs of the Foundation in accordance with the policies established by the House of Delegates.

After the reorganization, the Medical Administrative Committee was eliminated. These changes made a major difference in the relationship between the ARA Section representing the volunteer medical and scientific (research) arm and the predominately lay Board of Trustees. The ARA continued to have its own committee structure to serve its professional and scientific functions.

In 1979 Dr. Daniel McCarty, President of the ARA, recorded his thoughts about the "marriage" of that organization with the AF. His words also reflected the opinions of the majority of the ARA members. He wrote that since the reorganization "communication between lay and professional volunteers improved greatly but decisions and problems dealt with by AF committees now often bypassed ARA Executive Committee review completely. Medical policy evolved and promulgated by AF often had only nominal ARA input. These policies were sometimes presented to groups such as the National Arthritis Advisory Board (NAAB), the National Institute of Arthritis, Metabolism and Digestive Diseases (NIAMDD), and even congressional committees about the same time that the ARA leadership became aware of them. Some of the functions of the AF committees continued to overlap to a considerable degree with ARA committees (e.g., Professional Education). These problems have been largely remedied" (85). On the whole, he was of the opinion that the union was a stable one and that the appointment of Dr. Frederic C. McDuffie as Senior Vice President for Medical Affairs in 1979 had resulted in improvement in communications between the Foundation staff and the members of the ARA Section.

Progress in Government Relationships. During the past 35 years, the Foundation has worked closely with government at all levels: federal, state, and local. Within the federal government, arthritis research is conducted through programs of the National Institutes of Health (NIH), primarily through the National Institute of Arthritis, Diabetes, Digestive and Kidney Diseases. This Institute, created in 1950, spent $44 million on arthritis programs during 1982. Approximately another $15,000,000 for arthritis-related research was provided by other institutes, particularly the National Institute of Allergy and Infectious Diseases, the National Institute of Aging, and the National Institute of Dental Research.

In 1975 the Arthritis Act was passed by Congress and signed into law by President Gerald Ford. This action resulted from an intensive educational effort by the AF Government Affairs Committee under the Chairmanship of Mr. Porter Nelson, with the able assistance of Dr. Charley Smyth and Mr. Galen Broyles, all of Denver. This Arthritis Act provided for the appointment of an Arthritis Commission, which spent the next 12 months preparing a plan for action. This body was chaired by Dr. Ephraim Engleman of San Francisco. The nine members of this commission, which included representatives from academic rheumatology, rheumatologic practice, government, people affected by arthritis, and the public, conducted hearings in several cities throughout the country. Also, they reviewed voluminous amounts of written testimony as well as the recommendations of several task forces on areas such as education, research, patient care, and epidemiology.

In April 1976 their five-volume report was presented to Congress and the President. The report resulted in the establishment of a new NIH program, the Multipurpose Arthritis Centers (MACs), and some increase in the arthritis research budget. During the first six years (1977–82), the NIH funded 22 Multipurpose Arthritis Center Programs with grants totaling more than $32.8 million.

Increase in Services to Patients. As the Arthritis Foundation entered into its 35th year, bringing more and better services to patients and their families continued to be a major goal. The 71 local chapters and divisions bear the largest part of this responsibility.

It is at the community level that volunteers and local staff provide a wide variety of helpful programs. Many chapters sponsor arthritis clubs or support groups for individuals with specific diseases (such as juvenile arthritis and systemic lupus) to meet together and share personal problems and successes. People with arthritis can also take advantage of special activities conducted by chapters, such as the Arthritis Aquatic Program or other group exercise programs. Patient education is an important goal; chapters provide educational material, including pamphlets, films, slides, and reference resources. The

Arthritis Self Help Course is offered by many chapters; this six-week series of classes is designed to help its participants gain the knowledge and skills necessary for an active role in patient care.

Chapters also serve as important community information centers about the rheumatic diseases. Public forums are presented to inform the community of the various types of arthritis and ways to cope with the disease. Some chapters maintain a speakers bureau of volunteers, many of whom have personal experience with arthritis.

Other services include drug discount programs and loan closets of self-help devices and medical equipment. Each chapter maintains a referral list of physicians qualified to treat arthritis patients. Chapters frequently serve as centers for information about other medical and social service programs in the community. Home-visit programs sponsored by some chapters provide supportive listening, information about community services, assistance with self-help devices, and adaptation of the residence. Counseling services by professionals or trained volunteers who have arthritis are also available in many chapters.

American Juvenile Arthritis Organization. For many years arthritis in children remained a neglected subject. When rheumatic fever was common, children with other forms of arthritis were frequently given this diagnosis mistakenly. As streptococcal infections and their sequelae decreased, the existence of juvenile arthritis became more apparent. From the turn of the century to 1970, there was a widespread belief that juvenile rheumatoid arthritis was the same disease as adult rheumatoid arthritis and that the clinical differences simply reflected differences in the expression of the disease process in growing individuals. However, as a result of the observations of pediatric rheumatologists, especially in the United States and Britain, it became apparent during the late 1960s and 1970s that juvenile rheumatoid arthritis had at least three distinct forms and might not be a single disease. This new concept plus the gradual emergence of pediatric rheumatology as an important subspecialty and a recognition of the unique problems of children with arthritis led Clifford Clarke, President of the Arthritis Foundation, and Judith Smith, Vice President for Patient Services, to organize a small task force of parents. This group met in Atlanta in 1978 to consider what might be done to develop an organized attack on the problems of juvenile arthritis. Those attending this meeting were Mrs. Barbara Barrett of Seattle, Washington, Mrs. Arlene Johnson of Avon Lake, Ohio, and Mrs. Dawn Hafeli of St. Clair Shores, Michigan.

As a result of this meeting, Mr. W. W. Satterfield, Chairman of the Arthritis Foundation, appointed a Panel on Juvenile Arthritis to consider how the Arthritis Foundation could better focus on the unique needs of parents and children with rheumatic diseases. In April 1980 this Panel reported to the Board of Trustees that the public at large, academic institutions, and the government were generally unaware of the serious medical and socioeconomic problems presented by these children.

A few centers offering specialized care for children with arthritis and performing research had been established in the late 1930s and 1940s, including those at the Robert Breck Brigham Hospital in Boston, Presbyterian Hospital and Bellevue Hospital in New York, and Childrens Hospital in Los Angeles. Also, the American Rheumatism Association had established a Council on Pediatric Rheumatology in 1975 and in 1976 had sponsored an important conference on rheumatic diseases of childhood. Nonetheless, too little had been accomplished in the way of increased funding for research, training of fellows, or organized patient care. The Panel recommended that: 1) the Board of Trustees establish an organization within the Arthritis Foundation to counsel the Board of Trustees and the House of Delegates on matters relating to rheumatic diseases of children; 2) this organization provide channels for communication and cooperation among parents, physicians, and health professionals; 3) this organization develop and recommend to the Foundation and its chapters programs and activities to meet the needs of children affected by the rheumatic diseases. As a result the Board and subsequently the House of Delegates approved the establishment of the American Juvenile Arthritis Organization. Mr. Satterfield appointed a 12-member AJAO Executive Committee of parents and pediatric rheumatologists to elect its officers and establish its bylaws. In addition the AJAO was provided representation on the Board of Trustees and House of Delegates and the opportunity to nominate members to Foundation committees.

The first meeting of the Executive Committee was held in Cleveland in March 1981, at which time Mrs. Arlene Johnson was elected president. In November 1983 she was succeeded by Mr. Richard Weaver of Sacramento, California, and in 1984, Mr. Albert Moseke of Washington, DC, became president. A membership organization was established by the national office and a newsletter for parents has been distributed at regular intervals since that time.

A major activity of members of the AJAO has been to continue working with the federal office of Maternal and Child Health, particularly with Dr. Merle McPherson, to establish federally funded centers for pediatric rheumatology throughout the country. The first three centers funded in 1982 were in Houston, Texas (Dr. Earl Brewer), Philadelphia, Pennsylvania (Dr. Balu Athreya), and Los Angeles, California (Dr. Virgil Hanson). By 1984 the number of centers had increased to 11, in Denver, Washington, DC, Atlanta, Honolulu, Chicago, Kansas City and Omaha, New Orleans, Boston, Cincinnati, Philadelphia, and Houston. The funds for these centers, $120,000 to $150,000 each, have enabled them to improve their patient care activities by hiring additional health care personnel, such as nurses, physical therapists, occupational therapists, and social workers to help with the special problems of children with arthritis. In 1982 the Arthritis Foundation established the first Pediatric Clinical Research Center at the University of California in San Francisco headed by Dr. Arthur Ammann. By 1984 two additional centers, at Northwestern University and the University of Washington in Seattle, were funded.

The AJAO has worked closely with the Patient Services and Government Affairs Departments of the Foundation in developing programs and educational materials for parents and children with arthritis and with government agencies to secure the rights guaranteed to handicapped children by law.

In July 1984 the first parents' conference was held in Keystone, Colorado, under the leadership of Ms. Kathy Angel of Houston, Texas. In 1985 the Arthritis Foundation committed itself to hiring a full-time staff director for the AJAO. Thus, though growth has been frustratingly slow and at times erratic, the Organization has now clearly found an important niche within the Arthritis Foundation. It promises to provide increasingly important services for children with arthritis and their parents as well as stimulate opportunities for further research.

Major Emphasis on Changing Public Image of Arthritis. The Board of Trustees of the AF at its 1980 annual meeting adopted a plan to help bring about the Foundation's ultimate objective of finding the causes, the prevention, and the cure of arthritis. The top goal approved under this plan was to "create a presence of the AF nationally as a strong, dynamic, effective and credible organization." Among the strategies to be used to reach that goal were: 1) to develop sharply targeted advertising and public relations programs using modern marketing analysis methods; 2) to enhance the image of the Foundation in the eyes of the general public and members of the health professions by selecting and carrying out educational activities that would give wide exposure to programs and purposes of the Foundation.

This campaign is already showing results. More people know the facts about arthritis than ever before, but still the greatest problem in the fight against arthritis is public apathy. The theme of the public information campaign of the Foundation: "It's time we took arthritis seriously" will motivate thousands of our citizens to move toward a victory over arthritis.

9

Arthritis Health Professions Association

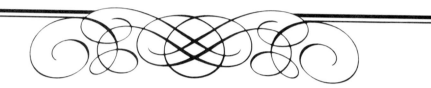

DURING the first 15 years of the Arthritis Foundation, there was rapid growth in the public awareness of the magnitude of the overall health problems and the economic burden caused by arthritis and related disorders. With this development came an increasing recognition of the importance of the contributions of many health disciplines in providing the full range of patient care to the millions in this country affected by arthritis.

To address this concern, in 1962 the Arthritis and Rheumatism Foundation provided a stipend of $250 to two national organizations, the American Physical Therapy Association and the American Occupational Therapy Association, to set up an advisory committee to the Foundation. Dr. William Clark, President of the Foundation, encouraged the inclusion of all allied health professionals who were involved in the care of people with arthritis.

Dr. Morris Ziff, temporary Chairman of the Medical Administrative Committee (MAC) of the Foundation, stated in a letter dated August 5, 1965, "With the amalgamation of the American Rheumatism Association and the Arthritis Foundation into one strong organization we have taken an important step in the fight against arthritis. The next step is to bring into the organization the talents of the many paramedical people throughout the country who have over the years demonstrated their interest in arthritis. To this end the by-laws of The Arthritis Foundation, approved by the Board of Directors on June 19, 1965 provide, under Article VI, Section 1D, for a Paramedical Section of the Medical Council" (150).

⊹ *EARLY YEARS (1965 to 1971)*

To establish this section, a planning commitee was appointed composed of Chairman, Dr. Joseph Levinson, from Convalescent Hospital for Children, Cincinnati, Ohio; Dr. Nadene Coyne, Director of Physical Medicine and Rehabilitation at Cleveland Metropolitan General Hospital; Edna Farrington, RN, of the Arthritis Clinic at Columbia Presbyterian Hospital in New York City; Jean Reid, RN, RPT, of the Southern California Chapter in Los Angeles; Marion Sutcliffe, a statistician from New York University Medical Statistics Unit; Elaine Terry, OTR, from the Dallas County Hospital District in Texas; and Addie Thomas, ACSW, Director of Social Work at Johns Hopkins Hospital in Baltimore, Maryland.

This group met October 1, 1965 to plan for the organization of a paramedical section. Forty interested persons, primarily from arthritis centers and representing a variety of allied health professions, gave thoughtful consideration and voted unanimously that a section be formed but raised objection to the term "paramedical." It was also strongly expressed that the organization not be fractionated by profession or into subgroups but that all members function and work together as in an ideal interdisciplinary clinical setting to effect a coordinated team pattern of interaction.

Purposes of the organization were set forth as: 1) the establishment of interdisciplinary communication about comprehensive services, teaching, and research in the rheumatic and connective tissue diseases; 2) the stimulation and promotion of ideas and activities within and among the respective disciplines in relation to these diseases; 3) the promotion of public understanding of comprehensive approaches to the care of persons with these diseases.

Thus "the Paramedical Section of the Medical Council of the Arthritis Foundation was organized by 40 charter members in 1965 and became official in June 1967 when its rules of procedure were ratified" (4). Elected as its first President was Addie Thomas, ACSW; Vice-President, Elaine Terry, OTR; Secretary, Jean Reid, RN, RPT. Others on the first Executive Committee were Joy Cordery, OTR, from the Institute of Physical Medicine and Rehabilitation in New York City, Martha Morrow, RPT, from Strong Memorial Hospital in Rochester, New York, and Berthold Wolff, PhD, a psychologist from New York University School of Medicine in New York City.

The Paramedical Section held its first and second Annual Membership and Scientific Meetings in June 1966 in Denver (during its de facto state) and June 1967. Although several of its committees were concerned with membership and organizational matters, the Paramedical Section Education Committee began work early on two important projects: drafting a booklet on home care in arthritis and a manual for nurses, physical therapists, medical social workers, and other associated health specialists. These projects were to be published and distributed by the Arthritis Foundation. In accordance with the expressed wishes of the organizing group and the membership, the name of the Section was changed in June 1968 to *Allied* Health Professions Section. In 1978 this Section became the *Arthritis* Health Professions Section. The present name, Arthritis Health Professions Association (AHPA), was adopted in 1980 to reflect the evolving professionalism and to parallel the name of the American Rheumatism Association (120).

Early membership was fostered by new educational programs funded with social and rehabilitation grants from the federal government. Between 1965 and 1973, membership increased to approximately 250 and, from 1973 on, rapidly escalated to 1800 by 1984.

This growth was attributed to the federal funding of Arthritis Regional Medical Programs in the early 1970s and the development of the NIH Multipurpose Arthritis Centers. Local AHPA sections in more than 26 states also contributed to this growth with new sections continually being organized (120).

Cross memberships on appropriate ARA and AHPA committees were initiated early by Dr. Donald Hill of Tucson, Arizona, who was Chairman of the MAC and President of the

American Rheumatism Association in 1966-67. The Allied Health Professions Section also had representation on the Medical Administrative Committee and on site visits for grant requests and reviews for centers.

Educational conferences were held regularly after the first meeting in 1966, which had been held in conjunction with the American Rheumatism Association. One panel in particular, on body image, generated much interest at that first meeting. These meetings were held semiannually. In 1970 the topic "Extending the Care of the Arthritis Patient into the Community" attracted many AHPs in Columbus, Ohio and then again in San Mateo, California in 1971. It was the forerunner of regional conferences that eventually replaced the midwinter semiannual meetings.

Although primarily oriented to education of its membership, AHPA early on was well aware of its deficits in research. In June 1968 the AHP Executive Committee moved that a Research Committee be added to its structure with the goal of promoting scientific methods and multidisciplinary research projects. More immediate goals were to suggest research activities and investigate the creation of a fellowship program. Dr. Joseph Levinson chaired this first committee. In 1970 the first AHP representative was appointed to the Arthritis Foundation Fellowship Committee.

MIDDLE YEARS (1972 to 1978)

In keeping with its mission of providing a forum for the sharing of clinical and research experiences, the Section also provided a quarterly newsletter to keep the membership informed of current events, educational tools, seminars, and reviews of the literature. The first issue, put out by Elaine Terry, appeared in February 1967. Eventually the newsletter responsibility was assumed by a Publications Committee, which was first chaired by Robert Richardson, RPT, in 1969-70. Joy Cordery, OTR, maintained this important function with dedication from 1971 to 1980.

This period also saw the *Home Care Manual*, begun earlier, disseminated by the Foundation and distributed to patients through physicians. The *Self-Help Manual* was developed by many AHPA members under the leadership of Judith Klinger, OTR as a comprehensive handbook for patients. It described more than 450 specific aids for daily living. A *"How-to"* Manual for Patient Education showed AHPs how to set up individualized educational objectives for patients. The task of compiling the *AHPA Teaching Slide Collection for Teachers of Allied Health Professionals*, which would eventually contain 198 slides and a syllabus, was begun.

The fellowship program for the training of nonphysician health professionals was established in 1973. The first three-year AHP fellow selected was Jeanne Melvin, OTR, MS, of the University of Southern California; she wrote and published *Occupational Therapy Guide for Treatment of Rheumatic Diseases* under the guidance of Dr. Robert Swezey. In 1974 the second fellowship was awarded to Joan Sutton, RN, MSN, from Johns Hopkins University in Baltimore to develop a university program in rheumatic disease nursing.

In 1975 there were 19 applications for three fellowships, which were awarded to: Louis Adams, BS, University of Cincinnati, for a pilot study of laboratory personnel as an AHP resource; Bozena Pietrzak vel Pietrowski, MSc, McGill University, Montreal, to develop a program for the training of a rheumatologist's assistant; and Pamela Rand, LPT, MS, of St. Margaret Memorial Hospital in Pittsburgh, to evaluate patient education programs in arthritis.

The tenth anniversary of the AHP Section in 1975 coincided with the creation of the national Arthritis Commission appointed by President Gerald Ford (see Chapter 10). In 1976 the Commission, in a report to the President, recommended an emphasis on the role of allied health professionals, patient education, and research in treatment, epidemiology, environmental, social and behavioral aspects of arthritis, and health services. The vehicles to carry out these recommendations were 24 multipurpose arthritis centers, which were funded in 1977 and brought many new allied health professionals not only into the centers but into the association. Meaningful research became more evident from the fellows and other members of the organization, and the quality of scientific content at meetings began to improve.

In 1978 the Arthritis Foundation began to fund AHP research grants with stipends of $3000. The first four recipients studied: identification of psychological stress as a risk factor in the flare of rheumatoid arthritis; effectiveness of an instructional program for patients with rheumatoid arthritis in an ambulatory setting; evaluation of the test-retest reliability of a functional assessment form; and the analysis of function in rheumatoid arthritis with finger joint replacement.

Although well on their way, the grant and fellowship programs were not without difficulties, including lack of research expertise by AHPs, poor dissemination of information to potential grant and fellowship applicants, and the need for guidelines in proposal preparations. In 1978 an AHP Executive Workshop in Research was held to address these problems, with the goals of improving quality and quantity of proposals, stimulating research, and training AHPs to take leadership roles in rheumatology.

RECENT YEARS (1979 to 1985)

During this period, the organization remained dedicated to providing educational opportunities for health professionals, especially those generalists who had little previous training in rheumatology and those arthritis specialists who could remain in rheumatology and ultimately train others. In 1980-81, for the first time, seminars were conducted in each of the four regions, allowing many members who could not attend a national meeting to participate in a rheumatology conference. Attendance at annual scientific sessions had increased significantly. In 1977, 250 AHPs attended the meeting in San Francisco. By 1981 470 participated in the Boston meeting, for which there was a 24% increase in submitted abstracts; also, participants at the Boston meeting had the opportunity, for the first time, of receiving AHPA continuing education units (120).

AHPA membership expanded to include more than 14 disciplines, including biostatisticians, dieticians and nutritionists, health educators, medical technologists, nurses, occupational therapists, orthotists, pharmacists, physical therapists, physicians, psychologists, research associates, social workers, vocational counselors, and others. Students in the health professions also became eligible for membership. In 1984 the Association included not only professional care providers but educators, researchers, and health care administrators, with 29% of its membership coming from the field of physical therapy, 26% from nursing, 20% from occupational therapy; 6% social work; 6% health education; 6% medicine; 4% rehabilitation counseling; 1% laboratory/medical work; and 7% from "other" disciplines including psychology and college administration. (The numbers equal 105% because some members fit into more than one category.) These professionals came from 47 states, all provinces of Canada, Australia, England, Northern Ireland, and Venezuela. Growth of AHPA membership is shown in Figure 9-1.

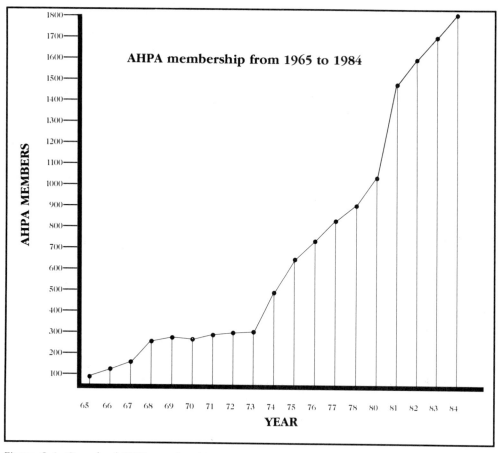

Figure 9-1. Growth of AHPA membership.

In 1980 the first research methodology workshop was held at an annual meeting, and emphasis shifted from developing new reseachers (a project that remains) to finding qualified researchers (52).

In 1981 stipends for research grants were increased from $3000 to a maximum of $15,000 to make these awards more meaningful. Combined Arthritis Foundation, AHPA fellowship and research grant awards increased from $78,500 in 1977 to $219,332 in 1984. (See Table 9-1.)

By 1985, 30 research grants and 31 fellowships had been awarded. All the fellows had remained active in the rheumatology field, and, indeed, all continued to be active in either the Arthritis Foundation, the Arthritis Health Professions Association, or both. The alumni of the fellowship program had an average of 8.2 publications per person and up to 21 scientific publications since completing their award periods. These individuals also contributed substantially to the literature of rheumatology and patient education materials. Several went on to advanced degrees, particularly doctoral degrees, and some received faculty appointments. All spent time in the areas of teaching, research, patient care, and administration with almost 40% of the time accounted for in research activity (53).

Table 9-1. Arthritis Foundation combined AHP Fellowship and Research Grant Awards

Year	Amount	Year	Amount
1977	$ 78,500	1981	172,000
1978	83,000	1982	132,542
1979	65,599	1983	202,187
1980	123,241	1984	219,332

Of particular note are a few research projects that have had significant impact. In physical therapy, Barbara Figley Banwell, RPT, MA, from the University of Michigan, looked at adapting exercise programs for the handicapped and studied aerobic exercise for cardiorespiratory training in patients with rheumatoid arthritis. Michael Rapoff, PhD, from the University of Kansas, was awarded a research grant to design an effective method to improve salicylate therapy compliance in children with arthritis. Shirley Sahrmann, PhD, from Washington University in St. Louis, examined the relationship of altered neuromuscular responses and knee joint pathology to overall function in patients with arthritis.

The most widely publicized project, by Kate Lorig, RN, DrPH, from Stanford University, was a randomized prospective study of the effects of patient education on people with arthritis. In her original study, 300 arthritis patients received 14 hours of training on the nature of arthritis, its management, and general principles of arthritis care, including medications and physical measures. The cost of this training was approximately $15 per person. The patients were trained by lay leaders, most of whom had arthritis. Leaders received prior training and were given specific information to relate to the patients. This program was field-tested in Arthritis Foundation chapters and Multipurpose Arthritis Centers around the country and then sponsored by the national office of the Arthritis Foundation to be disseminated to its 71 chapters.

In 1982 the AHPA annual scientific sessions were totally integrated for the first time with the American Rheumatism Association's at the Pan-American League Against Rheumatism Congress held in Washington, DC. Many members of ARA attended AHPA sessions and vice versa, and many combined workshops were held. This cooperation allowed both organizations the opportunity of sharing ideas.

A Committee on Affiliated Professional Sections was strengthened during this period with outstanding members from each of the four regions appointed by the President. The objectives of this Committee were to "assist in the development of local AHPA sections and offer guidance in strengthening those local sections already in existence, strengthen regional educational programs, and encourage more active participation of local section members in the activities of the Arthritis Foundation," (6) such as providing speakers for professional and public education programs, consultants to patient clubs, articles for chapter newsletters, and increased visibility of the AF chapter. The Arthritis Foundation's "Standards of Chapter Performance" required AHPA representation on all chapter committees. Guidelines for organization of local AHPA sections were available from the Arthritis Foundation to interested professionals. By 1984, there were 30 established local AHPA sections nationwide. Most worked closely with their local Arthritis Foundation chapters.

Rheumatology standards by the various nursing and allied professional groups began to be considered. Under the leadership of Janice Pigg, RN, BSN and Marie Heiss, RN, MS, standards for rheumatology nursing were established in conjunction with the American Nurses' Association and copublished under the title "Outcome Standards for Rheumatology

Nursing Practice." As the publication explains, "The standards offered in this document focus on patient outcomes and include rationales specific to individuals with rheumatic disease" (103).

The first AHPA review course at the annual scientific sessions (Anaheim, June 1985) was designed for interdisciplinary arthritis clinicians with an intermediate level of knowledge. After an update of current information regarding diagnosis and treatment of common rheumatic diseases, the course focused on in-depth knowledge and treatment of selected patient problems requiring interdisciplinary intervention.

Since rheumatology was not taught in many schools of nursing and allied health professions, AHPA established a subcommittee, chaired by Marjorie Becker, PhD, from the University of Michigan, to explore the development of a model rheumatology curriculum for use in nursing, physical therapy, and occupational therapy schools. Such a curriculum would also serve as a model for care of chronically ill persons and geriatric and disabled patients.

This period also saw efforts to foster international networking to disseminate the products and ideas of AHPA to other countries. By 1984 AHPA members were presenting papers at conferences in France, England, Germany, Australia, Canada, Mexico, and Denmark.

THE TWENTY YEAR MARK: FUTURE PROSPECTS

Although AHPA has experienced rapid growth over the past several years, its potential as a professional organization is still unknown. There are more than three million people in the nursing and allied health professions from whom to draw, and the leadership of AHPA today is focusing on what needs to be done.

Although it is essential to have excellent research to show that the methods AHPA members use in their practice are scientifically sound in changing the course of disease, improving function, or reducing overall costs (53), most members are practitioners outside the academic environments where research is traditionally done and do not come from training bases where research was emphasized. Consequently, research will continue to be a challenging priority that will involve the search for increased funding to develop a cadre of competent health investigators.

A survey of family and general practitioners and internists in Tucson, Arizona highlights a recurrent problem of the organization—that the roles of allied health professionals are misunderstood (121) and that the physician, other allied health specialists, and the public must be educated as to the role of each discipline. This education can be done by adding arthritis to nursing and allied health school curricula and by exposing medical students, primary care residents, and rheumatology fellows to arthritis health professionals during their training. Publication of journal articles describing AHPA disciplines and practice, and the development of standards of care are other ways to ensure the roles are well understood.

Most health professionals can define what a team should be and why it is particularly necessary in the care of the chronically ill arthritis patient, who may require multiple rehabilitative techniques. However, effective team functioning in the present health care system seems to evade practical application. Nurses and allied health professionals on the interdisciplinary team still must learn about the necessary ingredients for successful team operation: inclusion of the patient as an equal partner, sharing of knowledge, development of good communication skills, and dedication to a common goal.

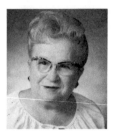
Addie G. Thomas,
L.C.S.W.B.
1966–68

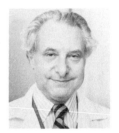
Berthold Wolff, Ph.D.
1968–70

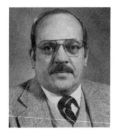
Ronnie E. Townsend,
M.P.H.
1970–71

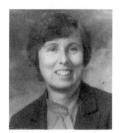
Phyllis Cohn Annett,
R.N., M.P.H.
1971–72

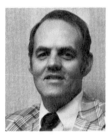
Marlin N. Shields, R.P.T.
1972–74

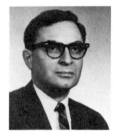
Max Weiner, Ph.D.
1974–75

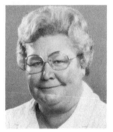
Marjorie C. Becker, Ph.D.
1975–76

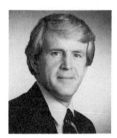
Robert W. Richardson,
L.P.T., M.Ed.
1976–77

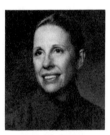
Janice Smith Pigg,
R.N., B.S.N.
1977–78

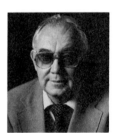
David Wayne Smith, Ph.D.
1978–79

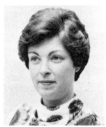
Joan D. Sutton, R.N., M.S.N.
1979–80

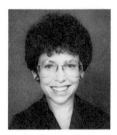
Gail E. Riggs, M.A.
1980–81

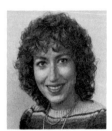
Julia W. Parker, R.P.T.
1981–82

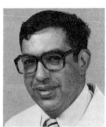
Eric P. Gall, M.D.
1982–83

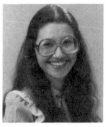
Colleen C. Miller,
R.N., M.S.N.
1983–84

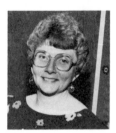
Barbara Figley Banwell,
M.A., P.T.
1984–85

Figure 9-2. AHPA Presidents, 1966 to 1984.

As a professional organization, AHPA is strong and getting stronger. Internally it has good communication and a sense of comraderie. The variety of disciplines represented in AHPA makes it a unique organization; the respect for this variety and willingness of many disciplines to work together make it an exceptional Association. The Arthritis Health Professions Association of the Arthritis Foundation is committed to research, education, and service providing growth opportunities to not only its members but the patients they're dedicated to serving.

10

Growth and Contributions of the National Institute of Arthritis and Metabolic Diseases

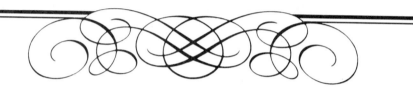

THE National Institute of Arthritis and Metabolic Diseases came into being with the Omnibus Medical Research Act passed by Congress and signed by President Truman on August 16, 1950, as recounted in Chapter 6. Like all the National Institutes, its programs included intramural research carried out in laboratories in the complex in Bethesda, Maryland and a much larger extramural program of grants-in-aid of research and training done in appropriate institutions throughout the United States. An immediate start was made with intramural research by continuing projects already in progress in laboratories of the Experimental Biology and Medicine Institute, which had merged with the new National Institute of Arthritis and Metabolic Disease.

Dr. William Henry Sebrell, Jr., who had directed the previous Institute since 1948, became the first Director of NIAMD. Only a year later, however, he was appointed Director of NIH as a whole and was succeeded at NIAMD by Dr. Russell M. Wilder on March 6, 1951. The latter, in turn, was succeeded as Director of NIAMD by Dr. Floyd S. Doft on October 1, 1953. Dr. Doft continued as Director for nine years and played an important role in this formative period. Dr. G. Donald Whedon was Director from 1962 to 1981, when he was succeeded by Dr. Lester B. Salans until 1984, when Dr. Mortimer B. Lipsett became Director.

Meanwhile, in July 1953 the large and well-equipped Clinical Center on the Bethesda site was opened, providing an immediate expansion of facilities for laboratory research and clinical studies and for the care of patients with arthritis and metabolic as well as other diseases. Dr. DeWitt Stetten, Jr. was appointed Director of Intramural Research to guide the expanding intramural program of basic research and clinical investigations. In 1954 Dr. Joseph J. Bunim left the Rheumatic Diseases Study Group at New York University to become the first intramural Clinical Director and Chief, Arthritis and Rheumatism Branch. He was responsible for clinical training and research in rheumatic diseases in the new Clinical Center. A rheumatologist of first rank, an inspiring teacher, and a dedicated clinical

DIRECTORS, NIAMD—NIADDK

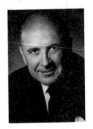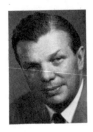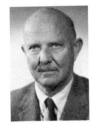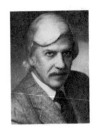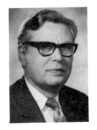

DIRECTORS, INTRAMURAL & EXTRAMURAL RESEARCH

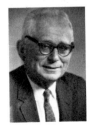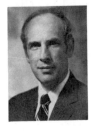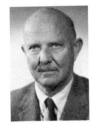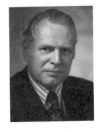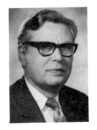

CHIEFS, ARTHRITIS AND RHEUMATISM BRANCH, INTRAMURAL PROGRAM

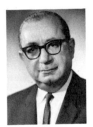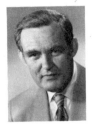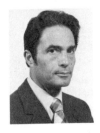

| DIRECTOR, DIVISION OF ARTHRITIS, MUSCULOSKELETAL AND SKIN DISEASES | CHAIRMAN, NATIONAL COMMISSION ON ARTHRITIS AND RELATED MUSCULOSKELETAL DISEASES |

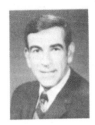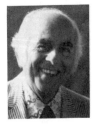

Figure 10-1. Directors of NIAMD and NIADDK. From left to right, Dr. William H. Sebrell, Jr., 1950-51; Russell M. Wilder, 1951-1953; Floyd S. Doft, 1953-62; G. Donald Whedon, 1962-81; Lester B. Salans, 1981-84. Directors of Intramural Research: DeWitt Stetten, Jr., 1954-74; Joseph E. Rall, 1974-83; Directors of Extramural Programs: Ralph E. Knutti, 1951-61; John F. Sherman, 1961-64; Ronald W. Lamont-Havers, 1964-72. Chiefs, Arthritis and Rheumatism Branch, Intramural Program: Joseph J. Bunim, 1954-64; John L. Decker, 1964-83; Henry Metzger, 1983—; Director, Division of Arthritis, Musculoskeletal and Skin Diseases: Lawrence E. Shulman, 1976—; Chairman, National Commission on Arthritis and Related Musculoskeletal Diseases: Ephraim P. Engleman, 1975.

investigator, he contributed greatly to the development of rheumatologic research at the Clinical Center in that early period and in the ensuing years until his untimely death in 1964 (Figure 10-1).

EXTRAMURAL PROGRAM

The extramural program of grants for research and training in institutions throughout the country expanded even more impressively. The principles governing this program of grants had been soundly laid under the guidance of Dr. Cassius James Van Slyke, who had joined NIH in 1946 as Chief of the newly established Research Grants Office, later renamed the Division of Research Grants. Final decisions regarding the fate of applications submitted for grants in the field of arthritis were made by the National Advisory Arthritis and Metabolic Diseases Council at their periodic meetings held in Bethesda. On the basis of previous review by appropriate study sections of NIH and Council members and by review at the Council's meetings, priorities were assigned to the approved applications, which were then awarded within the limits of the funds available. At the Council meetings Dr. Van Slyke impressed all with his breadth of vision and statesmanship.

Direct responsibility for the NIAMD's research and training grants was in the hands of Dr. Ralph E. Knutti, who was appointed chief of extramural programs of research grants, training grants, and fellowships in 1951 and, subsequently, Associate Director for Extramural Programs in 1960. He fulfilled these duties with skill for 10 years before being appointed Director of the National Heart Institute in 1961. He was followed by Dr. John Sherman until 1964, when Dr. Ronald Lamont-Havers became the new director. Dr. Lamont-Havers continued until 1972, when the Institute was reorganized on a divisional basis. Although a Division of Extramural Activities continued to provide services, many of the responsibilities for rheumatologic extramural programs became the province of the Division of Arthritis, Musculoskeletal and Skin Diseases.

On November 19, 1953 the First National Conference on Research and Education in the Rheumatic Diseases was held at the National Institutes of Health under the joint sponsorship of NIAMD, the American Rheumatism Association, and the Arthritis and Rheumatism Foundation (153). This conference brought together rheumatologic leaders from throughout the United States to discuss current research and education in the rheumatic diseases and point the way to promising avenues for future efforts (Figure 10-2). A second similar conference was held in 1957 (154), and others subsequently.

Program-Project Grants. In 1959 an important new development was launched with the establishment of program-project grants. Grants in support of individual research projects, although important, were of little help in creating rheumatologic units in medical schools. Sizable grants for programs rather than projects in cancer and heart disease had been made for some years through the national institutes concerned with those illnesses, but little support of this type was available for arthritis. The need for such support for rheumatology was particularly great. Although significant work in cancer and heart disease had been in progress in most medical schools even before the large grant support, similar programs in rheumatic diseases existed only at Harvard, Columbia, New York University, the University of Michigan, and the University of Pennsylvania, as discussed in Chapter 2. This need was particularly apparent to the members of the National Advisory Arthritis and Metabolic Diseases Council, who joined with Dr. Doft and his staff in urging Congress to include such funds in the appropriations for the National Institute of Arthritis and Metabolic Diseases. With the important support of Senator Lister Hill and Representative John Fogarty

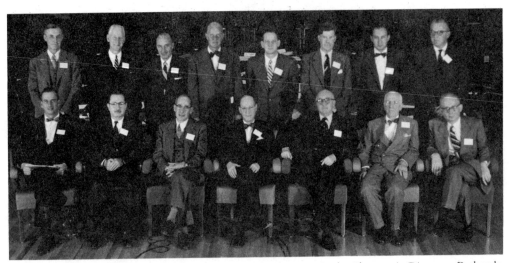

Figure 10-2. National Conference on Research and Education in the Rheumatic Diseases, Bethesda, Maryland, November 19, 1953. First row: Gideon DeForest, Joseph Bunim, Karl Meyer, T. Duckett Jones, Floyd Odlum, Russell Cecil, DeWitt Stetten, Jr. Second row: John Deitrick, Currier McEwen, Richard Freyberg, Ralph E. Knutti, Maclyn McCarty, Granville Bennett, Jerome Gross, Charles Ragan.

in their respective congressional committees and that of Mrs. Mary Lasker as a dedicated citizen (see Figures 6-1 and 6-2, pages 56 and 57), these efforts were successful.

By their very nature, applications for these large amounts required most careful evaluation, including an on-site visit by several experts in the appropriate fields of science and not merely study of a written application. A special Program-Project Committee was appointed within the framework of the National Advisory Arthritis and Metabolic Diseases Council to be responsible for the new program and to make its recommendations to the Council. The committee membership had to be large because the site visits to applicant medical schools would be made chiefly by members of the committee.

Dr. Currier McEwen, who as a member of the NIAMD Council had worked for the establishment of the new program, was appointed chairman of the Program-Project Committee with the following members: Drs. Robert R. Cadmus, Alexander B. Gutman, Thomas H. Hunter, Mr. Raymond W. Kettler, Drs. E. Henry Keutman, Henry D. Lawson, James E. McCormack, Albert I. Mendeloff, Carl R. Moyer, Donald Murray, William D. Robinson, William H. Sebrell, Jr., Joseph Stokes, Jr., and Louis G. Welt. Dr. Harold M. Davidson, from the Division of Research Grants, served as Executive Secretary.

A preliminary ad hoc planning committee meeting was held on May 27, 1961, and the first full committee meeting took place on September 29, 1961 with only three members absent. The first year only $200,000 in new funds was available, but the appropriations for this program increased yearly (Figures 10-3 and 10-4). Applications for grants poured in from medical schools, requiring considerable time and effort for site visits by the committee members, but the program was highly successful, and within a few years, significant rheumatologic units were developing throughout the United States.

It is of interest that after their eagerness to see this program established, the National Advisory Arthritis and Metabolic Diseases Council became concerned lest the program expand faster than trained, academically oriented rheumatologists would be available to lead the new units. Actually this expansion proved advantageous. Chairmen of departments of medicine who had wished to develop such units but lacked the necessary funds, now selected able young internists not already irrevocably committed to some other subspecialty and offered them these opportunities. The result was the infusion of a new generation of able young men and women into positions of responsibility and leadership, and the modern period of scientific rheumatology was well on its way.

INTRAMURAL PROGRAM

In 1974 Dr. DeWitt Stetten, Jr., left NIAMD and was succeeded as Director of Intramural Research by Dr. Joseph L. E. Rall, who served until 1983, when he was appointed Director of Intramural Research for NIH as a whole. He was replaced by Dr. Jesse Roth. After the death of Dr. Bunim in 1964, his two positions were separated. Dr. Robert S. Gordon, Jr. took over as Clinical Director, and in September 1965 Dr. John L. Decker joined the staff as Chief, Arthritis and Rheumatism Branch. Dr. Decker and Dr. Philip S. Gordon alternated as Clinical Director in the late 1970s and early 1980s until 1983, when Dr. Decker was appointed Director, Warren Grant Magnuson Clinical Center, leaving the organizational fold of NIADDK. Dr. Henry Metzger, a Senior Investigator of the unit, was appointed Chief, Arthritis and Rheumatism Branch.

Other scientific leaders of the intramural program included Dr. Leon Sokoloff, who was recruited from New York University by Dr. Bunim in 1953. He contributed greatly with his skills in experimental pathology over the years until he resigned in 1973 to become a professor of pathology at the State University of New York at Stony Brook. Similarly, Dr. J. Edwin Seegmiller contributed enormously with his studies on purine metabolism from 1949 until 1969, when he moved to the University of California, San Diego.

REORGANIZATION OF INSTITUTE

In contrast to the National Cancer and Heart Institutes, the National Institute of Arthritis and Metabolic Diseases was, from its start in 1950, concerned with several areas of medicine in addition to rheumatologic and metabolic illnesses. These areas included nutrition, dermatology, gastroenterology, hematology, renal diseases, and orthopedics. Subsequently, as Congress directed larger emphasis on gastroenterologic research, the name was changed in 1972 to the National Institute of Arthritis, Metabolism and Digestive Diseases. Reflecting expanding programs in diabetes and nephrology, the name was again changed in 1981 to the National Institute of Arthritis, Diabetes, Digestive and Kidney Diseases. This change did not result from lesser interest in rheumatologic diseases but emphasized the goals and responsibilities of the Institute as a whole and furthered its role in diabetes, gastroenterology, and renal diseases.

Also in accordance with these overall changes in the Institute, a reorganization was effected subdividing it functionally into six divisions: 1) Intramural Research; 2) Arthritis, Musculoskeletal and Skin Diseases; 3) Diabetes, Endocrinology and Metabolic Diseases; 4) Digestive Diseases and Nutrition; 5) Kidney, Urologic and Blood Diseases; 6) Extramural Activities. In 1974 Dr. Nancy B. Cummings was appointed Associate Director for Kidney, Urologic and Blood Diseases and Dr. Harold F. Roth, Associate Director for Digestive Diseases and Nutrition. Similarly in 1976, Dr. Lester B. Salans became Associate Director for Diabetes, Endocrinology, and Metabolic Diseases.

ARTHRITIS ACT

As mentioned in Chapter 8, a major purpose of the Arthritis Foundation has been to work closely with the United States Congress and state and local legislative bodies on matters relating to arthritis. One important outcome of these efforts was the national Arthritis Act of 1974, which was signed into law in January 1975. One of the provisions of the Act was the creation of the National Commission on Arthritis and Related Musculo-skeletal Diseases. Dr. Ephraim Engleman was appointed Chairman of the Commission and the members were Verna Patton Anthrop, BS, PHN, K. Frank Austen, MD, Rosalind Russell Brisson, William F. Donaldson, MD, William R. Felts, MD, Vivian Floyd Lewis, PhD, Doris Melich, Howard F. Polley, MD, Gordon C. Sharp, MD, Marlin N. Shields, RPT, and also distinguished representatives from the Veterans Administration, the Department of Defense, and various of the National Institutes of Health. Dr. William H. Batchelor, Special Assistant to the Director of NIADDK, served as Executive Secretary (99).

In April 1976, after a year of study and public hearings, the Commission issued its report to Congress, the Arthritis Plan (97). This Plan contained 145 recommendations based on analysis of major areas such as research, education, care of patients, and community concerns. Specifically the Plan called for increasing arthritis research and training, undertaking epidemiologic studies and establishing data systems in arthritis, establishing a National Arthritis Information Service, creating multipurpose arthritis centers throughout the United States, and appointing a National Arthritis Advisory Board.

The first such Board was established in 1976, with Dr. Engleman as chairman. In July 1976 Dr. Lawrence E. Shulman relinquished his leadership of the rheumatology program at the Johns Hopkins University School of Medicine to become Associate Director of NIADDK in charge of the program concerned with arthritis, bone, and skin diseases and to help create and implement the Arthritis Plan presented to Congress that year. Under his leadership, many of the recommendations of the National Commission were initiated, including the establishment of an Office of Epidemiology and Data Systems, the Arthritis Information Clearing House, an Arthritis Interagency Coordinating Committee, the National Arthritis Advisory Board, and a series of multipurpose arthritis centers across the country. In 1983 the rheumatologic aspects of the NIADDK were raised to divisional status when the Division of Arthritis, Musculoskeletal and Skin Diseases was created, with Dr. Shulman as its head.

OTHER PROGRAMS

In addition to the programs previously mentioned, NIADDK developed and supported various other activities, including epidemiologic studies, a program of rheuma-tologic research in cooperation with the USSR, a systematic program of studies through a cooperating group of clinics in the United States, and the development of the multipurpose arthritis centers.

The epidemiologic studies, under the direction of Dr. Peter H. Bennett, were begun in 1960 among Blackfoot and Pima Indians in Montana and Arizona. These studies led to the establishment of a center in Phoenix, Arizona for epidemiologic and clinical studies of osteoarthritis and rheumatoid arthritis in southwestern Indian populations.

Scientific cooperation with the USSR was encouraged by "scientific exchanges" sponsored by the two governments. Through these programs, selected groups of laboratory and clinical specialists visited research institutions in the other country to compare methods and exchange ideas. The exchange sponsored by the NIAMD was made up of men representing the various medical subspecialties of concern to that Institute. Dr. William Henry Sebrell, Jr., former Director of the Institute and also of NIH, served as scientific leader of the team of six, and Dr. Floyd Doft, then Director of NIAMD, was responsible for administrative details. Dr. Currier McEwen represented rheumatology, Dr. William B. Castle, hematology, Dr. Clifford J. Barborka, gastroenterology, and Dr. J. Murray Luck, a biochemist, served as interpreter.

The Russian team came to the United States in 1959, and the United States group also scheduled its tour for that year. However, the day before they were to leave, word was received from the Russian Embassy postponing the trip for a month. Most members of the United States team could not reschedule their teaching commitments and the visit, therefore, was postponed until the fall of 1960. Dr. Castle, unfortunately, could not be free at that time and had to withdraw. In the USSR the team participated as a whole in the formal activities, but each member devoted most of his remaining time to institutions and departments in his subspecialty. During the week in Moscow, therefore, most of Dr. McEwen's time was spent at the Institute of Rheumatism directed by Academician A. I. Nesterov, who was also generally responsible for the program in rheumatology throughout the USSR (87).

A second visit sponsored by NIAMD in 1964 concerned only rheumatology. Its members were Dr. Joseph Bunim, Chief, Arthritis and Rheumatism Branch of NIAMD, Chairman; Drs. Ronald Lamont-Havers, then Medical Director of the Arthritis and Rheumatism Foundation, Gene H. Stollerman, John H. Vaughan, and Morris Ziff.

In 1972 the United States signed an agreement with the USSR for a cooperative program of research in arthritis, the fourth such major collaboration in the health sciences between the US and the USSR. The first meetings of the American and Russian scientists under this program were held in Moscow in January 1974; there, preliminary decisions were reached regarding cooperative studies to be undertaken. Large clinical trials of D-penicillamine were carried out on patients in Moscow and New York; retrospective studies of children with juvenile arthritis were also performed. Other cooperative studies included the treatment of nephritis of systemic lupus, the establishment of criteria for assessing progressive systemic sclerosis, the development of specific measures of functional disability in patients with rheumatoid arthritis, and the evaluation of endoprosthetic replacement in orthopedic operations for arthritis.

One of the other important programs of the NIADDK was the sponsorship and support of statistically sound evaluations of various therapeutic measures by a group of cooperating clinics organized by the American Rheumatism Association in the early 1960s in response to the prodding and leadership of Dr. Donald Mainland of New York University. Subsequently, these studies were developed under contract with the University of Utah under the direction of Dr. John Ward. In 1977, as mandated by the Arthritis Act, the American Rheumatism Association Medical Information Service (ARAMIS) was established at Stanford University Medical Center under the direction of Dr. James Fries.

Useful as the various miscellaneous activities developed and supported by NIADDK are, the programs of most importance have been the fundamental ones of intramural research at the Bethesda campus and, especially, those of extramural support of research and education at medical schools throughout the United States. The NIADDK has also supported research in other countries if appropriate to the nature of the health problem under study.

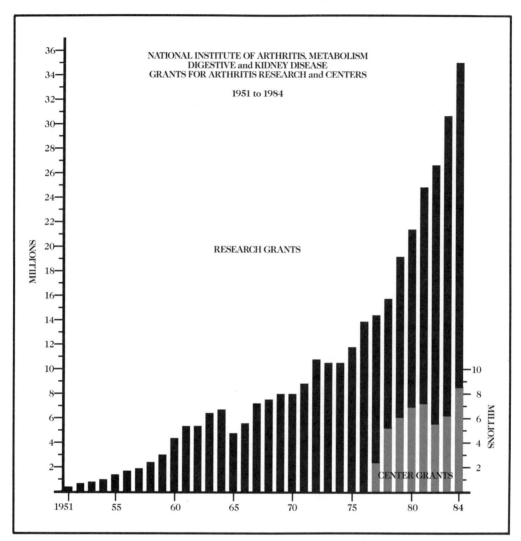

Figure 10-3. NIAMDDK. Grants for Arthritis Research and Centers, 1951-1984.

GROWTH IN FUNDS

The growth in the funds appropriated for arthritis and other rheumatic diseases between 1951 and 1984 is illustrated in Figures 10-3 and 10-4, which represent the NIADDK allocations for research and multipurpose arthritis centers and for training grants and fellowships in rheumatology (42). Table 10-1 summarizes the allocations since 1972 for arthritis and other concerns of the Division of Arthritis, Musculoskeletal and Skin Diseases compared with the total for all disease categories of the NIADDK. Funds for arthritis and related disorders in 1981 accounted for only approximately 12% of the total NIADDK budget, but these funds made a threefold increase during this nine-year period of growth.

Particularly worthy of comment is the excellent spirit of mutual cooperation that has existed from the start among the National Institute, the American Rheumatism

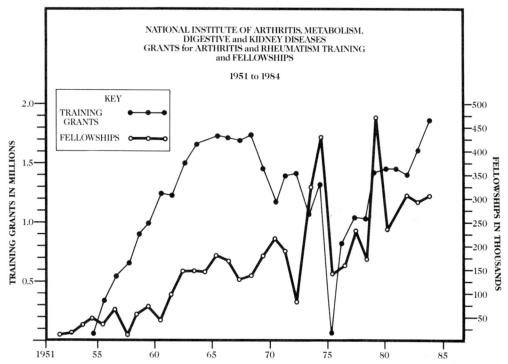

NATIONAL INSTITUTE OF ARTHRITIS, METABOLISM,
DIGESTIVE and KIDNEY DISEASES
GRANTS for ARTHRITIS and RHEUMATISM TRAINING
and FELLOWSHIPS

1951 to 1984

Figure 10-4. NIAMDDK. Grants for Arthritis and Rheumatism Training and Fellowships, 1951-1984.

Table 10-1. NIADDK Program Funding, 1972 to 1984

	Division of				
Year	Arthritis and Related Disorders	Musculo-skeletal	Skin Diseases	Total	Total All NIADDK Programs†
1972	14.4*	5.8	4.9	25.1	139.6
1973	13.8	5.6	4.7	24.1	134.9
1974	14.1	6.0	5.0	25.1	147.9
1975	16.9	7.6	4.8	29.2	167.0
1976	19.1	8.2	4.8	32.1	175.0
1977	23.3	9.4	6.1	38.8	211.0
1978	27.9	10.5	7.5	45.9	249.4
1979	33.8	12.6	8.8	55.2	291.2
1980	37.4	14.7	9.1	61.2	327.2
1981	43.2	16.3	10.2	69.8	356.2
1982	42.9	16.7	9.7	69.3	353.8
1983	48.1	17.8	11.9	77.8	397.9
1984	55.1	20.2	12.8	88.1	464.6

* Dollars in millions.

† Totals may be inexact due to rounding.

Association, and the Arthritis Foundation. This cooperation has been aided by representation of leaders from each organization serving on committees, boards, and councils of the others but is chiefly due to a true spirit of common interests and purposes. The relationship over the years has been a remarkable example of partnership, informal but no less real, between a governmental agency, a professional society, and a voluntary fundraising foundation, all collaborating without friction and with mutual confidence and esteem in their efforts for the conquest of one of mankind's most serious ills.

11

Progress in the Management of Rheumatic Diseases

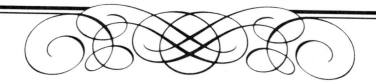

EXCEPT for the discovery of the value of colchicine in the treatment of "rheumatism" in the sixth century AD and salicylates in the late 1800s, essentially all the progress in the treatment of rheumatic diseases has taken place since the 1930s. The advances have included a number of true therapeutic triumphs but in the most important forms of arthritis have consisted of measures that are ameliorative rather than curative. In this chapter, the extremely important therapies that have led to cure or control are discussed first, and the treatment of rheumatoid arthritis is then considered in greater detail to exemplify the developments in the treatment of arthritis in general.

Before taking up these individual measures, however, mention must be made of two developments fundamental to any rational approach to treatment, namely, the establishment of a classification and of diagnostic criteria for the major forms of rheumatic diseases, and the use of statistically valid methods in appraising results. In the United States, both these developments stemmed from efforts of the American Rheumatism Association (see Chapter 7). Although the use of drugs to lessen pain could be helpful in all types of arthritis, any reasonable efforts to develop measures directed at pathogenesis required some understanding of the various forms of articular diseases. Much remains to be learned about the basic mechanisms of most rheumatic diseases, but the establishment of a classification and diagnostic criteria was an important first step.

Before the development of statistically sound means of evaluation, trials of new measures and medications were subject to bias by the physician and the wishful thinking of the patient. The introduction of trials to compare the effect of the drug under study with that of a placebo without the patient knowing which he was receiving marked one step. However, it soon became apparent that the unconscious or even conscious bias of the physician was also a cause of error. From this experience came the "double-blind" clinical trials in which a third person, usually a statistician, codes the trial drug and placebo and neither the patient nor the physician knows which is being taken until the end of the study. For such dramatic therapeutic effects as those of salicylates in rheumatic fever and penicillin in pneumococcal pneumonia, the double-blind trial was scarcely necessary to reach valid conclusions. Unfortunately, most therapeutic results are not that striking, and acceptable conclusions can be reached only by precise, statistically sound evaluations of suitably large numbers of patients with well-defined diagnoses.

The Therapeutic Triumphs

Although opinions may differ on what should be included in a list of therapeutic triumphs, few would disagree with including 1) the prevention of rheumatic fever, 2) the cure of bacterial infections of joints, 3) the discovery of cortisone, 4) the treatment of systemic lupus erythematosus, 5) the control of gout, and 6) surgical replacement of damaged joints. These advances are presented in chronological order.

ADVANCES IN UNDERSTANDING AND PREVENTION OF RHEUMATIC FEVER

In the later 1800s astute clinicians had observed that attacks of rheumatic fever were frequently preceded by tonsilitis and scarlet fever (23). With the subsequent recognition that hemolytic streptococci caused those diseases, physicians speculated that these bacteria might also be involved in rheumatic fever. In 1931 the studies of Coburn focused attention on this possibility (25), and in the following year this concept received strong support from immunologic evidence showing the presence of a hemolytic streptococcal antitoxin (antistreptolysin-O) in the sera of most patients with rheumatic fever (152). These antibodies were present whether or not a preceding streptococcal infection had been observed, thus supporting the view that such infections were essential in causing the disease even when so mild they escaped clinical recognition. However, some patients failed to show any measurable increase in antistreptolysin-O, and the possibility therefore remained that other microorganisms might also cause the disease.

These observations regarding hemolytic streptococci led to a new era of intensive research, stimulated during World War II by outbreaks of rheumatic fever in recruits brought together in military camps. As noted in Chapter 2, extremely important studies were carried out in the streptococcal research laboratory at the Warren Air Force Base Hospital in Cheyenne, Wyoming under the direction of Dr. Charles H. Rammelkamp, Jr., which added much new knowledge of the epidemiology of rheumatic fever (115). Evidence rapidly accumulated that left no doubt that rheumatic fever could be induced only by a pharyngeal infection with group A hemolytic streptococci (144). This finding explained only part of the pathogenesis of the disease, leaving as yet uncertain the means by which the infections invoke rheumatic fever. However, this discovery did provide important information needed to devise methods to treat and prevent the inciting hemolytic streptococcal throat infections through use of antibiotics (3). As a result, rheumatic fever, which was formerly a cause of acute polyarthritis and serious heart disease, is no longer a significant problem in the United States, although it continues to be serious in areas of the world with inadequate medical care, malnutrition, overcrowding, and poor sanitation.

In contrast to the effective measures to prevent rheumatic fever, the treatment of existing disease has seen no sharp improvement since the introduction of salicylates in 1876

(80,118,145). Corticosteroids, which were hoped to be curative, probably are effective only in lessening inflammation and pain, like the salicylates, and do not alter the course of rheumatic carditis (156-158). They do, however, suppress fever and other features more rapidly than do salicylates and hence may be life saving in fulminating cases. The outlook for patients with chronic heart failure from rheumatic valvular disease has significantly improved through advances in cardiac surgery.

THE CURE OF BACTERIAL INFECTIONS OF JOINTS

No advance in the treatment of arthritis has been so striking or effective as that of the cure of bacterial infections of joints by appropriate antimicrobial agents. Before the introduction of the antibiotics, such infections as gonorrhea, pneumonia, sepsis, tuberculosis, and syphilis were common. Because of the lack of effective treatment, their complications, including joint infection, were also frequent. Patients with supurative infections of joints were common on the wards of general hospitals, remained for months, and invariably were discharged with badly damaged joints.

The first effective antibacterial agents developed for clinical use were the sulfonamides. In 1935 Domagk reported that the azo dyes, prontosil and neoprontosil, were strong antibacterial agents, particularly against streptococci (36). Other and better sulfonamides soon became available.

The greatest advance in antimicrobial therapy came in 1941 with the demonstration by the Floreys (45) that penicillin, which had been discovered by Fleming in 1929 (44) but not put to practical use, was an extremely potent bacteriocidal agent. With the discovery of streptomycin (133) and subsequently of isoniazid (123) used with para-aminosalicylic acid, highly effective treatment of tuberculous infections became available. The advent of penicillin led to intensive and successful efforts to discover other antibiotics with broader spectra of effectiveness. The primary infections promptly became curable in most instances, resulting in far fewer articular complications; when such sequelae did occur, they in turn could be successfully treated.

THE DISCOVERY OF CORTISONE

No doubt everyone interested in arthritis and rheumatism through the past 35 years knows the dramatic story of cortisone. The following account focuses attention on events before and after the announcement by Dr. Philip S. Hench of the discovery of cortisone, made in April 1949. Much of this story was related by Dr. Hench himself in remarks made in May 1953 (60).

In April 1929 Dr. Hench observed a patient with rheumatoid arthritis who had a remarkable remission when he developed jaundice. During the next five years, he saw this happen 15 more times. He speculated that an "antirheumatic substance X" developed during liver disease with jaundice. In the 1930s Dr. Hench and others studying arthritis repeatedly observed remission of rheumatoid arthritis in women during pregnancy. Could the unknown "substance X" of pregnancy be the same as that of jaundice? He suspected the mysterious substance was neither a product of the liver nor a female hormone but possibly a hormone common to both sexes.

At this point Dr. Hench sought chemical expertise, especially from Edward C. Kendall, PhD, Chief of the Division of Biochemistry in the Mayo Clinic, who had isolated various compounds from the adrenal cortex. Several of these compounds were administered to volunteers with rheumatoid arthritis by Dr. Hench and his associate Dr. Charles Slocumb. None produced clinical benefit.

In the 1930s other biochemists including Dr. Thadeus Reichstein in Switzerland began isolating compounds from the adrenal cortex, but in only minute amounts, too little for clinical trials. It became obvious that to have sufficient amounts for adequate clinical trials it would be necessary to synthesize those compounds from bile—an extremely difficult undertaking. However, the task was taken up by Dr. Kendall and his associates and by research chemists of Merck & Co. Finally in May 1948, using methods "devised chiefly by Kendall and Dr. Lewis H. Sarett of Merck & Co.," the company had a few grams of 17-hydroxy-11-dehydrocorticosterone, a substance made from bile, designated "Compound E" by Dr. Kendall. Drs. James Carlisle and Randolph Major of Merck & Co. sent some of this compound to Dr. Hench in September 1948. Drs. Hench, Slocumb, and Polley began administering Compound E to a volunteer rheumatoid arthritis patient in September 1948. The antirheumatic effect "was unlike that of any previous remedy or of any condition except pregnancy or jaundice," according to Dr. Hench (60).

A few months later, Dr. John Mote of the Armour Laboratories provided Dr. Hench with another hormone that other scientists had isolated from the pituitary gland—the adrenocorticotropic hormone (ACTH). When injected into a patient with rheumatoid arthritis, this hormone produced effects similar to those of Compound E. In March 1949 Drs. Hench, Slocumb, and Polley received from Dr. Harold Hailman of the Upjohn Company enough of another adrenal cortical compound, Kendall's "Compound F" (hydrocortisone), to use in one patient for two weeks. Its effects were comparable to those of Compound E and ACTH.

Through the winter of 1948-49, the Mayo investigators injected Compound E into patients with rheumatic fever, systemic lupus erythematosus, hay fever, and "three or four" other diseases and were happy to note the results (60).

Consultants and staff of Merck & Co. required testing Compound E in other parts of the country before any announcement of the Mayo results. Accordingly, Dr. Hench invited five American investigators of rheumatic diseases to the Mayo Clinic to examine their studies: Drs. Walter Bauer, from Boston, Edward Boland, from Los Angeles, Richard Freyberg, from New York City, Paul Holbrook, from Tucson, and Edward Rosenberg, from Chicago. In only five days at the Clinic, the visiting physicians witnessed the effects of Compound E in two rheumatoid arthritis patients. All observers were amazed at what they saw. The clinical demonstrations and record reviews completely convinced each of the visiting investigators of the remarkable antirheumatic effects of Compound E, Compound F, and ACTH.

Merck & Co. supplied each of the five physicians enough Compound E to administer to two patients for two weeks in his own locality. Each participant was asked to report his findings independently in discussion of the paper to be presented by Dr. Hench and associates at the Seventh International Congress on Rheumatic Diseases the following June in New York City.

A few weeks after this "preview," late in April 1949, the cortisone studies were presented by Drs. Hench, Kendall, Slocumb, and Polley (Figure 11-1) for the first time at a scheduled meeting of the Mayo Clinic staff (62). The story appeared in the *New York Times* just after the staff meeting and immediately received wide attention and acclaim as a major

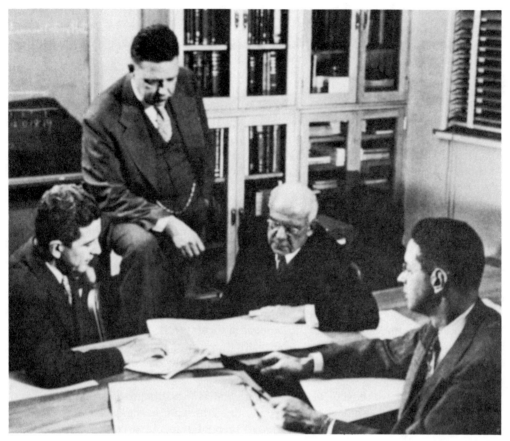

Figure 11-1. The cortisone team in 1949. From left to right, Charles Slocumb, Philip Hench, Edward Kendall, and Howard Polley. (From *Mayo Clinic Proceedings* 51:472, 1976)

contribution to the knowledge of rheumatism. Seven weeks later, the demonstration before the Seventh International Congress on Rheumatic Diseases (63) brought worldwide recognition of this important development. Nothing before or since had made such a tremendous impact on general interest in rheumatology or on the progress of research on rheumatic diseases.

Although Dr. Hench emphasized this research was being reported not as a new treatment but as a study of human physiology, the therapeutic implications were immediately recognized by the medical profession and many arthritis sufferers. Physicians wanted to obtain Compound E (cortisone) and Compound F (hydrocortisone, later cortisol) for therapeutic and investigational use. The demand could not be met; production was limited by the quantity of bile available and the technical difficulties of partial synthesis. Merck & Co. and other pharmaceutical manufacturers worked diligently to increase production, but supplies did not become sufficient to meet the demand until a new and larger source of the basic steroid structure to use as a starting material was found in yams and later, techniques were developed for the complete synthesis of cortisone.

Clinical investigators worked hard to determine the best therapeutic use of cortisone. Significant early research demonstrated that cortisone was effective when administered orally and Dr. Joseph Hollander's studies (71) showed hydrocortisone was beneficial locally when injected into the joints.

Unfortunately it soon became apparent that the tremendously beneficial antiinflammatory effects of cortisone were coupled with potentially serious undesired effects, including weight gain and abnormal fat distribution, osteoporosis, enhancement of infections, steroid myopathy, and emotional lability. Hence, although extremely valuable in life-threatening situations and for short-term administration in less serious rheumatic problems, long-term use of cortisone can lead to severe problems. Numerous analogs of cortisone and hydrocortisone were made by several pharmaceutical manufacturers in an effort to increase therapeutic effectiveness and eliminate, or at least diminish, undesired reactions to cortisone.

In 1954 prednisone and prednisolone became available to Dr. Bunim and his associates at the National Institute of Arthritis and Metabolic Disease. Dr. Bunim reported (18) that these analogs were three to four times more effective than cortisone milligram for milligram and that some undesired effects, especially those related to sodium retention, occurred less frequently. Soon thereafter, it was found that introduction of fluorine at the C9 position enhanced the effect of prednisolone; this discovery led to the production of new analogs, triamcinolone and dexamethasone. Although the newer analogs are effective in smaller doses, the undesired effects also appear at those levels.

The complete cooperation of the pharmaceutical manufacturers and the clinical investigators in rheumatology is nowhere more strikingly demonstrated than in this cortisone story.

Although the discovery of cortisone and ACTH and their antiinflammatory and antirheumatic effects was indeed a therapeutic breakthrough, its significance extends far beyond that. The importance is really threefold: 1) the therapeutic uses of the drug, 2) the broad scientific impact of the finding on medical research, and 3) the tremendous stimulus this discovery provided to the entire campaign against rheumatism. The potent antiinflammatory effect of the corticosteroids far exceeds that of any other therapeutic agent. This effect accounts for their widespread usefulness in the treatment of rheumatic diseases and many other illnesses.

The discovery of cortisone profoundly influenced scientific medicine and medical research. It pointed up the central position to rheumatology of many other medical fields—biochemistry, metabolism, and endocrinology. It led to research into the mechanism of inflammation, the role of immunology, genetics, and biochemistry in the rheumatic diseases, and it sparked many other studies of the etiology and pathogenesis of arthritis. The discovery gave rheumatologic research sparkle and attractiveness that stimulated many young investigators to apply their skills in this medical field.

The discovery could not have come at a more opportune time for the campaign against rheumatism in the United States. The cortisone story drew widespread public attention to arthritis and rheumatism as a public health problem, which strengthened the position of the infant Arthritis and Rheumatism Foundation and influenced Congress to establish the National Institute of Arthritis and Metabolic Diseases. These effects of the discovery of cortisone were discussed in detail in Chapter 5.

That the discovery of cortisone was an extremely important medical advance is further attested to by the award to Drs. Hench, Kendall, and Reichstein of the Nobel Prize in Physiology and Medicine in December 1950, less than two years after the first report was presented.

TREATMENT OF SYSTEMIC LUPUS ERYTHEMATOSUS AND OTHER LIFE-THREATENING CONNECTIVE TISSUE DISEASES

Before 1948 the diagnosis of systemic lupus erythematosus was entirely dependent on the presence of the clinical features of the disease, and the disease was frequently misdiagnosed except in acutely ill patients with the characteristic butterfly facial rash and high fever. In that year the situation was changed by Hargraves' discovery of the lupus erythematosus (LE) cell phenomenon in the blood of patients with the disease (58). These cells were subsequently shown to be neutrophils that have phagocytosed a homogenous mass of altered nuclear material extruded from another cell damaged by antinuclear antibodies. Thus in 1964, systemic lupus was found to belong in the category of autoimmune diseases (75). Eventually, techniques for measuring antibodies to various nuclear components improved the sensitivity and reliability of diagnostic tests. Physicians learned that the acute fulminating cases previously recognized made up only a relatively small segment of patients with the disease and that in many patients, the course tended to be chronic, with involvement of multiple organs and punctuated by occasional episodes of greater or lesser intensity. Meanwhile, with the availability of the corticosteroid drugs (62), and the use of other measures, it became possible to control the acute lupus crisis and improve survival. Thus the concept of systemic lupus and its prognosis has changed profoundly.

Although advances in the treatment of most of the other serious connective tissue diseases have been less dramatic than those for systemic lupus, the corticosteroids have also been helpful in treating vasculitis, polymyositis, and polyarteritis nodosa. The antihypertensive drugs, most notably captopril, have been life saving in patients with the severe and rapidly fatal renal involvement of progressive systemic sclerosis (scleroderma) (165). A dramatic change has also occurred in the previously rapidly fatal course of Wegener's granulomatosis through treatment with cyclophosphamide (31).

CONTROL OF GOUT

Colchicine, or crude preparations made from several species of colchicum, had been used in medicine since the time of Hippocrates, but no specific mention of this substance's use in gout has been discovered earlier than that of Psychriste, a physician attached to the court of the Byzantine ruler, Leon the Great, in the fifth century AD (54). The drug probably did not come into general use until the middle and later 1800s with the reports of Alfred Baring Garrod (54). Certainly, it has provided effective treatment of the acute, painful attack for the past hundred or more years.

Only recently, however, has there begun to be understanding of the mechanism of action of colchicine in relieving the acute gouty attack. In 1967 Malawista (83) showed that one action of colchicine is to suppress the release of lysosomal enzymes from the polymorphonuclear leukocytes. Other effects of the drug include interference with microtubular function of cells and inhibition of mediators of inflammation (82).

In spite of the effectiveness of colchicine in relieving the inflammation and pain of acute gout, it always had some disadvantages because of the narrow margin between therapeutic and toxic doses. Therefore, the introduction of the newer nonsteroidal antiinflammatory drugs, beginning with phenylbutazone in the early 1950s (166) followed by indomethacin and others in recent years, has been an advance in treatment of the acute attack. Colchicine, because of its apparent selective action in gout, gives some diagnostic aid that the newer drugs lack, but this is of minor importance since other and more definitive diagnostic methods are available.

Unfortunately for the victims of gout over the past hundred years, colchicine has no effect on lowering the serum urate level. Ending the acute episode, important as it was for relief of pain, did not prevent further attacks. Thus the life story of the gouty subject was one of recurrent painful episodes and gradual accumulation of urate deposits in the tissues as disfiguring tophi, resulting in progressive articular damage and sometimes secondary infection and renal failure. Fortunately this situation was changed in 1950 with the introduction of the uricosuric agent probenecid (56) and later by that of the potent xanthine oxidase inhibitor allopurinol (131). Both these valuable agents have the capacity to reduce the gouty patient's urate levels to normal. Although the patient's basic metabolic defect remains, the acute attack can usually be quickly controlled and further attacks prevented. As an added dividend to gouty individuals, most of whom are fond of food and drink, the rigid dietary restrictions formerly imposed are now rarely necessary.

This brief account of the important advances in the treatment of some of the rheumatic diseases covers only a few of the measures that have been used over the years in the care of patients with the various forms of illness affecting the joints. The remainder of this chapter is devoted to a chronologic discussion of these treatments. Rheumatoid arthritis is considered as a prototype disease in the discussion, but many of the therapies have been used equally in others of these illnesses.

Historical Summary of Measures Used in the Management of Rheumatoid Arthritis

The vast array of mostly ineffective, often highly fanciful, and frequently harmful forms of treatment in the early decades of the twentieth century was satirized by Dr. Russell Cecil in an alphabet of arthritis therapies, beginning with A for aspirin, B for bee venom, C for climate, D for diathermy, and concluding with Z for zero therapy (Do nothing!) (Figure 11-2) (20). In the following historical summary of treatment, a number of these measures that were worthless or harmful are mentioned as well as those having value, but not all in Dr. Cecil's alphabet were widely enough used to merit attention.

Developments in the management of rheumatoid arthritis are considered here under four main headings: 1) treatments used in the hope of curing the disease, 2) those for the suppression of inflammation and relief of pain, 3) measures to correct or prevent deformities and restore function, and 4) psychosocial aspects of treatment. In the earlier periods, the therapeutic measures advocated were rarely subjected to controlled evaluation and hence tended to be based on individual judgments. In the absence of statistically sound evaluation, worthless remedies often were continued for many years before their lack of value became recognized. Only since the 1950s with the advent of the double-blind clinical trial have new measures been systematically subjected to sound appraisal (Table 11-1).

A THERAPEUTIC ALPHABET FOR RHEUMATOID ARTHRITIS

Aspirin   **B**ee venom   **C**limate   **D**iathermy

Exercises   **F**ever therapy   **G**old salts   **H**ydrotherapy

Iron   **J**oint surgery   **KI**   **L**ow-calory diet

Massage   **N**eo-salvarsan   **O**rthopedics   **P**sychotherapy

Questionable methods   **R**est   **S**pas, sulphur   **T**ransfusions

Ultraviolet light   **V**accines, vitamins   **W**eight regulation   **X**-ray therapy

Young & Youman's lodoxyl   **Z**ero therapy (Do nothing!)   **&** (and-so-on)

Figure 11-2. Russell Cecil's Alphabet of Therapy for rheumatoid arthritis.

MEASURES FOR CURING THE DISEASE

Miscellaneous Treatments. It is difficult to be certain whether such measures as bloodletting and purging used in the middle ages through the nineteenth century were considered curative or merely ameliorative. Probably their most enthusiastic advocates considered them cures. By the mid to late 1800s, these treatments were clearly in disfavor. Drugs popular during that period included antimony and calomel as purgatives and opium and Dovers powders for pain. Other treatments widely used were sulfur and camphor baths, visits to spas, and, with the development of electricity, electromagnetism. Interestingly, acupuncture also had advocates in the mid-1800s (91). Faith in these measures was never very strong, and by the close of the century, the emerging sciences of bacteriology and immunology showed the inappropriateness of bloodletting.

Removal of Foci of Infection and the Use of Vaccines. Unfortunately, the birth of bacteriology resulted in another period of therapeutic errors with the concept of focal infection as the cause of arthritis. As noted in Chapter 1, this theory advanced by Billings (13) was rapidly and almost universally accepted not only in this country but also in Europe until the 1930s. The number of teeth, tonsils, and even gall bladders and other suspected "foci" removed because of this erroneous theory is incalculable. Along with the extraction of the suspected foci was the use of vaccines, either "stock" vaccines prepared by commercial laboratories or so-called autogenous ones prepared from bacteria isolated from the patient's own suspected focus. Even the most respected rheumatologists of the day, including such scientifically oriented physicians as Russell Cecil and Philip Hench, followed the trend. Only at the academically founded rheumatologic units at Harvard, Columbia, New York University, and the University of Michigan was the theory significantly doubted and

Table 11-1. Chronologic listing of developments in treatment of rheumatic diseases

Dates*	Drug or Procedure	Purpose	Current Status
Middle ages to 18th century	Blood letting and purges	To cure disease	Not used—a fallacy
1876 to present	Salicylates	To relieve inflammation	Very valuable—a milestone
1884 to 1920	Antipyrene	To relieve inflammation	Not used
1887 to 1970	Phenacetin	To relieve inflammation	Little use
1899 to present	Aspirin	To relieve inflammation	Very valuable
1912 to 1940	Removal of foci of infection	To cure disease	Not used—a fallacy
1915 to 1940	Vaccines	To cure disease	Not used—a fallacy
1915 to 1940	High colonic irrigations	To cure disease	Not used—a fallacy
1917 to 1935	Colloidal sulfur	To cure disease	Not used—a fallacy
1927 to 1934	Aminopyrine	To relieve inflammation	Not used
1929	Discovery of penicillin		A milestone
1929 to present	Gold salts	To control rheumatoid arthritis	Valuable
1931 to present	Understanding of rheumatic fever	To control rheumatic fever	Very important—a milestone
1935 to present	Sulfonamides	To prevent rheumatic fever	Very valuable—a therapeutic triumph
1935 to 1948	Massive doses of vitamin D	To cure rheumatoid arthritis	Harmful—a fallacy
1941 to present, with periodic revisions	Adoption of classification	To diagnose diseases	Very important—a milestone
1943 to present	Use of penicillin	To prevent rheumatic fever and cure infections	Very valuable—a milestone

* Some dates are approximate

those measures rejected. Because of these doubts, removal of foci and injection of vaccines slowly declined, although they continued to be fairly widely used throughout the 1930s. The controlled trials of vaccines by Dawson and Boots (32) proved their lack of value.

Colloidal Sulfur. From 1917 to 1938 colloidal sulfur was advocated in the treatment of rheumatoid arthritis by many clinicians but was considered of no value by at least as many and gradually ceased to be used (51).

Massive Doses of Vitamin D. Like most diseases, rheumatoid arthritis has at times been unscientifically linked to deficiencies of various vitamins. Lack of solid evidence of such a relationship prevented the widespread use of vitamins in arthritis except as a general supportive measure. However, 1935 saw the start of another therapeutic error after a report of benefit from massive doses of vitamin D (37). For some 10 years, this form of treatment received considerable attention but gradually was discredited as lacking significant benefit and causing hypercalcemia with potentially serious side effects (50).

The Slowly Acting Antirheumatic Drugs. This group of drugs, also known as remission-inducing drugs and disease-modifying drugs, has no immediate or direct effect on inflammation or pain but appears to affect some underlying mechanism of the disease. The group includes a number of gold compounds, several antimalarial drugs, D-penicillamine, immunosuppressive drugs, and perhaps others.

1944 to present	Streptomycin	To cure tuberculous arthritis	Very valuable
1948 to present	Knowledge of rheumatoid factors	To diagnose rheumatoid arthritis	Very important—a milestone
1948 to present	LE cell	To diagnose systemic lupus erythematosus	Very important—a milestone
1949 to present	Cortisone	To relieve inflammation	Very valuable—a milestone
1950 to present	Phenylbutazone	To relieve inflammation	Valuable
1950 to present	Probenecid	To control gout	Very valuable—a milestone
1951 to present	Intraarticular corticosteroids	To relieve inflammation	Very valuable
1951 to present	Immunosuppressive drugs	To induce remission in rheumatoid arthritis	Valuable
1951 to present	Antimalarial drugs	To induce remission in rheumatoid arthritis	Valuable
1952 to present	Isoniazid	To cure tuberculous arthritis	Very valuable
1957 to present	Sulfapyrizone	To control gout	Useful
1960 to present	Statistical methods	To evaluate drugs	Very important—a milestone
1960 to present	Total joint replacement	To restore function	Very valuable—a milestone
1961	Understanding of crystal-induced arthritis	To understand disease process	Very important—a milestone
1963 to present	Indomethacin	To relieve inflammation	Very valuable
1963 to present	Newer NSAIDS*	To relieve inflammation	Very valuable
1963 to present	Allopurinol	To control gout	Very valuable—a milestone
1964 to present	D-penicillamine	To induce remission in rheumatoid arthritis	Valuable

* NSAIDs—nonsteroidal antiinflammatory drugs; see Table 11-2.

Chrysotherapy. The first report of a trial of gold in rheumatoid arthritis was that of Lande in 1927 (77) who considered it useful in 14 patients. The greatest stimulus to interest in gold salts for rheumatoid arthritis was the report of Jacques Forestier in 1929 (46). Gold compounds had been thought useful in the treatment of tuberculosis, and because Forestier interpreted some features of the two diseases as similar he tried them in rheumatoid arthritis and noted benefit. On a visit to the United States in 1934, Forestier reported his results at a number of rheumatologic centers and the following year summarized his experience with gold in the first publication on the subject in this country (47). Since then gold therapy has been extensively accepted.

Despite many laboratory studies of its effects, its mode of action remains unknown. Unfortunately, treatment with gold salts is ineffective in 30% or more of patients with rheumatoid arthritis, and its frequent toxic effects, some potentially serious, further limit its applicability. Nevertheless, a number of carefully controlled therapeutic trials have given evidence of its value in patients with progressive disease that fails to respond to more conservative measures (30,38–40,48,162). Thus gold is an example of an agent first chosen for fallacious reasons but that is beneficial although its mode of action remains unknown.

Antimalarials. In 1951 Page (104) reported his experience with the synthetic antimalarial drug mepacrine in the treatment of 17 patients with discoid lupus. The cutaneous lesions improved strikingly as did those of his one patient with systemic lupus. He also mentioned that in two of his patients, "associated changes of rheumatoid arthritis" disappeared as the skin condition improved. Subsequent reports confirmed the value of the synthetic antimalarial drugs in improving the cutaneous lesions of both discoid and systemic lupus and as disease-modifying drugs in rheumatoid arthritis. Because the first antimalarial drugs had the undesirable effect of turning the skin yellow, they were gradually replaced by chloroquine and later by hydroxychloroquine. Many rheumatologists believe the antimalarials to be somewhat less effective than gold in rheumatoid arthritis, but the controlled multicenter evaluation by the Cooperating Clinics Committee of the ARA found these two groups of drugs similar in effectiveness (81).

D-Penicillamine. The third of these so-called disease-modifying drugs, D-penicillamine, came into use in the 1960s after the report of Jaffe (72). Its effectiveness as a sulfhydryl reducing agent that lowers the titer of serum rheumatoid factor in vitro suggested to him that the drug might ameliorate the disease. He used it with success and numerous reports have confirmed his findings.

Unfortunately gold, hydroxychloroquine, and D-penicillamine are not effective in all patients. Their mode of action is not known. They seem to help in about 70% or less of patients, some of whom experience full remissions. Since failure of one of these drugs does not necessarily mean failure of all, a second may be tried if the first is unsuccessful.

Unfortunately, it was soon learned that all three have the potential to cause serious undesirable reactions. For gold and D-penicillamine, these reactions include potentially severe dermatitis, bone marrow depression, and renal impairment; therefore, all patients on these regimens must accept the annoyance and expense of frequent blood and urine tests in addition to close clinical observation for other toxic features. Until recently a drawback of gold therapy was that patients had to be willing to undergo weekly intramuscular injections; subsequently, however, effective oral preparations were developed. Oral gold preparations have yet to be approved for use in the United States (as of March 1985). Hydroxychloroquine and D-penicillamine are taken by mouth. The significant, though rare, untoward effect of hydroxychloroquine is eye lesions, so patients taking this drug must have their eyes examined every three to six months. Another limitation of these three groups of drugs is that patients who benefit from their use are prone to undergo relapses of the disease after the treatment is discontinued. Nevertheless, in spite of their shortcomings, they do lead to improvement in a substantial number of patients and are the first drugs proved by careful, statistically controlled trials to have this capacity.

Immunosuppressive Drugs. Immunosuppressive drugs, also known as cytotoxic and antimetabolic agents, were introduced as chemotherapeutic agents for the treatment of cancer, but they were tried in rheumatoid arthritis and systemic lupus even before the role of immunologic mechanisms in those diseases was understood (34). Subsequently several studies supported their value in rheumatoid arthritis, including a multicenter, double-blind trial carried out under the auspices of the ARA (29). The chemotherapeutic drugs include alkylating agents (nitrogen mustard, chlorambucil, cyclophosphamide), purine and pyrimidine antagonists (6-mercaptopurine, azathioprine), folic acid analogs (methotrexate), and others. Because of their toxicity, these agents are primarily given only under careful controlled conditions and only to patients with extremely severe disease. In such selected patients who have failed to respond to other measures, they are often of definite value. Unfortunately, these drugs can cause bone marrow depression and probably increase the risk of developing certain types of malignancy, especially lymphoma.

Corticosteroids. When Hench and his colleagues (62) first reported the dramatic relief of pain, swelling, and stiffness experienced by rheumatoid arthritis patients after taking cortisone, this finding aroused hope that at last a cure for the disease had been discovered. It was soon learned, however, that cortisone and its analogs, although extremely powerful antiinflammatory drugs, were not curative and, furthermore, that continued use was associated with serious undesired effects.

Synovectomy. The surgical procedure for removal of the diseased synovial lining of the joints, once considered a locally curative measure, is discussed later in this chapter.

MEASURES TO SUPPRESS INFLAMMATION AND RELIEVE PAIN

The Salicylates. Not until 1876, with the discovery of salicylates, were there any effective drugs for the relief of inflammation and pain of rheumatoid arthritis. In that year three independent therapeutic trials of salicylates were reported. In the English-speaking world, MacLagan, from England, is usually credited with the discovery of the value of salicylates in the treatment of "acute rheumatism" (80). However, two German reports appeared that same year (118,145). Salicylic acid had been under study as an antipyretic in several German universities (119), and its use by Riess and Stricker was based on reasonable pharmacologic observations.

In contrast, MacLagan's reasons for choosing a salicylate seem rather whimsical by modern standards and provide interesting insight into one of the theories of drug action of that day, namely, the Doctrine of Signatures. According to this concept, one should seek a medicine for a given disease by testing plants that seemed to have something in common with the disease. At that time it was believed that acute rheumatism, as rheumatic fever was then called, occurred in people exposed to damp environments. MacLagan, therefore, turned to the willow tree as the source for a curative medicine because it grows in wet places (126). Like Forestier's reasons for trying gold in rheumatoid arthritis, MacLagan's premises were wrong, but the salicin extracted from the bark of the willow proved wonderfully helpful in relieving the severe pain and high fever of his patients.

The need felt by physicians for a drug that would relieve rheumatic pain is apparent by the speed with which the salicylates were tested in many countries. A number of confirmatory reports appeared in *The Lancet* and the *British Medical Journal* within a few months of the reports by MacLagan. The first American articles, stimulated chiefly by the reports from Germany, also appeared in 1876 (114,138).

In 1899 synthetic acetylsalicylic acid (aspirin) was introduced and has been the principal form of salicylate used since that time. Indeed, because of its value, not only in rheumatic diseases but also in reducing fever and relieving headache and the discomfort associated with upper respiratory tract infections and other illnesses, it has long been the most widely sold drug throughout the world. More than 30 tons are currently taken daily in the United States alone. Its more recently discovered effectiveness in lessening the tendency to intramusuclar blood clotting in patients with arteriosclerosis and coronary heart disease has resulted in a further increase in its volume of use.

The pharmacologic action of the salicylates has been the subject of innumerable studies, but the mechanism of their beneficial effects remained unexplained until the important research on prostaglandins by John Vane in 1971 (161). Since then, most of the analgesic and antiinflammatory effects of the salicylates are believed to result from inhibition of cyclo-oxygenase, a key enzyme in the pathway through which arachidonic acid is converted to prostaglandins.

It is extraordinary that, despite its obvious and dramatic antiinflammatory action in rheumatic fever, most physicians, before 1965, believed aspirin merely analgesic in chronic forms of arthritis. Those rheumatologists with experience in the care of patients with rheumatic fever as well as rheumatoid arthritis were well aware of its antiinflammatory property, but this knowledge did not become generally appreciated until the report by Fremont-Smith and Bayles in 1965 (49).

The success of aspirin stimulated the pharmaceutical industry to seek other antirheumatic drugs. In the early decades of this century, antipyrine and then cinchophen and neocinchophen enjoyed transient popularity that declined when further experience showed their toxic effects were more pronounced than those of aspirin and that they were probably slightly less effective (15). Aminopyrine was advocated by Schottmüller in 1927 (134), and its effectiveness in small doses was confirmed (136). It gave promise of being superior to aspirin until it was demonstrated by Kracke and Parker to cause agranulocytosis in susceptible individuals (74). Later experience showed this effect to be one of the potentially serious toxic effects of gold, D-penicillamine, and other drugs that have continued to be administered in spite of that hazard. However, in the case of aminopyrine, the report of Kracke and Parker made a dramatic impact on medical acceptance and the drug was quickly abandoned.

Corticosteroids. The discovery in 1949 of the extraordinary antiinflammatory effectiveness of cortisone has been discussed in Chapter 6 and earlier in this chapter. Although corticosteroids are the most powerful of all antiinflammatory drugs, their value is profoundly limited in rheumatoid arthritis and other chronic diseases by their untoward effects.

In 1951 Hollander and his associates (71) reported the special value of corticosteroids injected intraarticularly. Only hydrocortisone derivatives were found locally palliative in this way, and relatively insoluble esters of these were developed to increase duration of local effect. A single injection of 1 ml or even less of prednisolone tebutate or triamcinolone hexacetonide can suppress local inflammation for weeks or months, and such treatment can be repeated as needed. This method of giving corticosteroids, like systemic administration, does not cure the disease, but properly administered in suitable patients, it gives significant relief of inflammation and pain in the joints injected without the hazard of untoward effects associated with systemic treatment. Intraarticular injections are, of course, most feasible when only one or a few joints are the major site of inflammation.

Newer Nonsteroidal Antiinflammatory Drugs. The first of what may be considered the newer nonsteroidal antiinflammatory drugs, and the first since aspirin to remain in continued use, was phenylbutazone (Butazolidin), which was introduced in the 1950s. Its toxic effects, which include agranulocytosis, unfortunately, limited its value, but it continues to be useful, under careful clinical and laboratory monitoring, especially in patients with ankylosing spondylitis, gout, or tendinitis who do not respond well to other drugs. Indomethacin (Indocin), introduced in the early 1960s (137), proved to be a valuable addition to the ranks of antiinflammatory agents and was especially useful in the same diseases helped by phenylbutazone. Chiefly because it is more easily tolerated, indomethacin tended to replace phenylbutazone.

The success of indomethacin and the experience gained by attempting to produce more effective and less troublesome corticosteroids stimulated the pharmaceutical firms to develop new and better antiinflammatory drugs in the years after 1960. A partial list of the formidable array available in 1983 is shown in Table 11-2, and the number increases steadily. All can cause undesirable effects, some of which, such as gastric distress and rashes, tend to occur in varying degrees in most of the drugs. Certain reactions are drug-specific, such as the headaches and psychotropic effects some patients experience from indomethacin.

One might reasonably expect that in the proper therapeutic doses, all these agents would be comparable in relieving inflammation and pain in most patients with a given disease and, indeed, that all would be similarly effective in different diseases. Experience has shown, however, that such is not the case, for some of the nonsteroidal antiinflammatory drugs are particularly helpful in one or another of the rheumatic diseases and individual patients tend to respond better to one than to others. Thus, physicians have realized the advisability of trying several of these agents in succession to discover which is most suitable for a given patient. All of these drugs, like aspirin, appear to exert their analgesic and antiinflammatory effects mainly by inhibition of prostaglandin synthesis. In general all are comparably effective in appropriate doses, and the chief advantages of some are their lesser likelihood of causing gastric distress and their ease of administration. The half-life of aspirin, ibuprofen, phenylbutazone, and indomethacin is relatively short, so the drugs must be taken three or four times daily and their full effect does not continue all night. The benefit of others, however, lasts for 12 to 24 hours, so only one or two doses are required in a 24-hour period. To overcome the need for repeated doses of aspirin and indomethacin, modified forms have been prepared that need to be taken only morning and night. One disadvantage of the newer nonsteroidals compared with aspirin is their higher cost per effective dose. Unquestionably progress has been made since the reports of 1876, but the important breakthrough occurred then and the improvements since have been chiefly in achieving lesser gastric irritation and improving convenience of administration.

Other Measures for Relief of Pain.

Analgesic Drugs. All the drugs mentioned in the previous section, with the exception of the corticosteroids, have analgesic as well as antiinflammatory action. Additional analgesia may occasionally be desired for short periods even for patients with rheumatoid arthritis but more often for those with pain caused by disabilities related to trauma. Narcotics such as morphine that have strong addictive potential obviously have no place in the treatment of patients with chronic, nonterminal illnesses. Codeine and several recently developed narcotics that are less addictive are sometimes used, as is the non-narcotic analgesic acetaminophen (e.g., Tylenol), but since these drugs lack antiinflammatory action their role in the inflammatory forms of rheumatic diseases is relatively small.

Nonmedicinal Measures. In addition to the relief of pain and stiffness given by the antiinflammatory drugs, physical measures have been developed over the years. Belief in the healing effects of mineral springs goes back to ancient times, the Roman baths, and the earlier religiously oriented medical shrines of Greece and Egypt. Surely heat and massage were used in those ancient health centers to free contracted joints. Subsequently, the spa played an important role in the treatment of many different types of illnesses, especially in European countries. In the United States many thousands of patients visit Hot Springs in Arkansas, Saratoga Springs in New York, and other similar resorts.

By the mid-1900s there was little confidence in the curative value of the waters themselves. However, the total regimen of rest and freedom from stress combined with

Table 11-2. A partial list of nonsteroidal antiinflammatory drugs

Salicylates	*Propionic acid derivatives*
*Aspirin	*Ibuprofen (Motrin, Bufren)
*Numerous other salicylates	*Naproxen (Naprosyn)
*Diflunisal (Dolobid)	*Fenoprofen calcium (Nalfon, Fenopron)
Indoles	Flurbiprofen (Froben, Ansaid)
*Indomethacin (Indocin, Indocid)	Ketoprofen (Alrheuma, Orudis)
*Sulindac (Clinoril)	Fenbufen (Cinopal, Lederfen)
*Tolmetin (Tolectin)	Carprofen (Ridamyl)
Pyrazoles	Pirprofen (Rengasil)
*Phenylbutazone (Butazolidin)	*Phenylacetic acid derivatives*
*Oxyphenbutazone (Tandearil)	Fenclofenac (Flenac)
Azapropazone (Rheumox)	Diclofenac (Voltaren, Voltarol)
Feprazone (Methrazone)	*Pyroxicams*
Fenamates	*Piroxicam (Feldene)
*Mefenamic acid (Ponstel)	Isoxicam (Maxicam)
*Meclofenamate sodium (Meclomen)	
Flufenamic acid (Meralen)	
Tolfenamic acid (Clotam)	
Clofenamic acid	

* Approved for use in the United States as of 1982. From *Primer on the Rheumatic Diseases,* ed. 8. Atlanta, Arthritis Foundation, 1983.

heat, massage, and other physical therapy measures enhances the various other treatments prescribed by the spa physicians.

From the earliest times the spa physicians were bound to have a particular interest in arthritis because of the many patients with those illnesses who sought their help. That interest is well illustrated by the fact that the International League Against Rheumatism, the first organization formed to combat the rheumatic diseases, was founded through the efforts of spa physicians, as discussed in Chapter 3. Although physical therapy measures were important early in the care of arthritis patients in hospitals, the development of departments of physical medicine came more slowly. At the Hospital for the Ruptured and Crippled in New York (now The Hospital for Special Surgery), the first in that city devoted chiefly to the care of crippled patients, physical measures formed the basis of therapy from its founding in 1863 but a formally organized department of physical therapy was not established until 60 years later.

Other nonmedicinal forms of treatment have included acupuncture, a variety of electrical appliances, and such psychologically associated measures as biofeedback. Although acupuncture was mentioned in this country in the mid-1800s, it received little attention until recent years with renewal of visits by Americans to China. This attention led to a flurry of interest, and physicians and technicians trained in acupuncture techniques appeared in cities throughout the United States. However, experience has failed to show evidence that it can alter the course of arthritis, and no specificity for the location of the needles has been found (116,148).

The use of various "machines" to produce galvanic and other electric currents enjoyed great popularity in the 1800s with the rapid expansion of uses of electricity. As with the so-called health foods today, many of the advocates of these electrical treatments were sincere, but much of the promotion continued long after the usefulness had been disproved and verged on quackery. Indeed, various types of electrical or "nuclear" gadgets advertised today are outright quackery (see Chapter 8).

With the development in this century of the specialty of physical medicine and rehabilitation, the use of the physical techniques has been placed on a rational basis, evaluated by carefully controlled appraisals. Various electrical and other means of providing relaxing heat to stiff, painful soft tissues are not only helpful in relieving pain but also make the patient more able to carry out the therapeutic exercises in treatment, as discussed below.

MEASURES TO CORRECT DEFORMITIES AND TO RESTORE FUNCTION

This section is chiefly concerned with the role of the orthopedic surgeon in the correction of existing deformities but will also consider the measures of physical medicine essential in preventing disabilities and assuring success of the surgeon's efforts.

Since the days of the ancient Egyptians, heat and massage have been used with benefit, not only to relieve pain but also to help maintain function. Since the 1930s it has been increasingly realized, however, that the most important contribution of physical medicine to the patient with arthritis is a suitably planned and supervised program of therapeutic exercises. Hot baths or heat applied in other ways assist in relaxing painful, stiff muscles and other connective tissues, in stretching contractures, and in enabling the patient to follow the exercise program. It is the exercises themselves, however, that effect valuable benefits. It has been demonstrated that exercises, combined with splinting, can help prevent deformities and also correct them if not too advanced. For more severe deformities and for damaged joints, surgical procedures are required, and the advances made by orthopedic surgeons, particularly since 1960, have been among the most important contributions in the history of rheumatic diseases.

Early Orthopedic Developments. The first operative interventions in the treatment of diseased joints for trauma or infections surely were performed even before the first recorded instances during the early Renaissance. Reports of arthrotomy, or surgical opening of a joint cavity, for purulent joint swelling appeared in the literature in the later half of the nineteenth century (11). Understandably, however, operations of this type had little role in the days before the discovery of general anesthesia and aseptic techniques. During the 1880s, as a consequence of the introduction of the carbolic acid spray technique of antisepsis by Joseph Lister (1827-1912), surgeons began to think of supplementing arthrotomy with medications injected into the joints using such materials as iodoform and bone charcoal. In 1910 Beck (10) injected a mixture of bismuth and petroleum jelly, and later Murphy injected formaline in glycerine into patients with acute septic arthritis (95). As might be expected, these primitive attempts to eliminate intraarticular infections were not successful. In fact, no significant progress in overcoming bacterial infections was made until 1935 when Domagk (36) introduced the sulfonamides. Improved sulfonamide derivatives rapidly followed, and then at the outbreak of World War II came the epoch-making demonstration by the Floreys (45) of the tremendous potency of penicillin.

Resection of Joints. This operative procedure was used during the later half of the eighteenth century in the hope of avoiding the then-common practice of amputation for intractable joint infections. Credit for introducing the resection of joints into general surgical practice goes to Syme (1799-1870), the great Edinburgh surgeon, whose comprehensive book, *The Excision of Diseased Joints,* was published in 1881. Undoubtedly, most of the joints he excised were the site of infection, especially of tuberculous nature. Rheumatoid arthritic joints probably were rarely operated on in those days. According to Bick (11),

131

J. C. Warren of Boston performed a resection of an elbow joint in 1834, probably the first in the United States. The procedure was next done by Bigelow, also of Boston, who in 1852, reported the removal of the head of the femur in a 10-year-old boy with a septic hip joint (12). Meanwhile the American discoveries of general anesthesia by chloroform in 1842 and ether in 1846 had started to revolutionize surgery by permitting the surgeon to work slowly and carefully and to develop new and more meticulous operations. Today, resections of large joints have become obsolete, except as part of total joint replacement operations, but removal of metatarsal heads remains a satisfactory procedure to relieve the pain and deformity of the foot in rheumatoid arthritis.

Synovectomy. Removal of the diseased lining membrane of joints was one of the types of surgery that could be attempted after the introduction of anesthesia. Volkmann in Germany is reported to have used synovectomy in 1877 for tuberculous arthritis (1). Muller in 1884 appears to have been the first to perform the operation in the treatment of rheumatoid arthritis (93), and Schüller followed in 1887 (135). Goldthwait (55) probably was the first to perform a synovectomy in the United States and was followed in 1916 by Murphy (96), who operated on two patients with hypertrophic villous synovitis. It was the report of Swett (147), however, in 1923 that brought the procedure into more general use in rheumatoid arthritis. The term "prophylactic synovectomy" reflected the concept that the operation should be performed early to prevent rheumatoid damage to the joint.

Synovectomy enjoyed modest popularity for some 15 years but then fell out of use, only to be resumed again in the 1960s. The resurgence of interest in the operation is illustrated by the fact that more than 200 articles on the subject were published throughout the world between 1960 and 1982, most of them favorable. Unfortunately, only a few trials have been controlled, and these found the procedure disappointing. In a controlled multicenter trial of the operation (5), pain and swelling were somewhat improved for a year or two, but thereafter little difference was seen between surgically treated joints and control joints. The study concluded that synovectomy can be helpful in the selected rheumatoid joint but does not prevent recurrences and has little place in the overall treatment of the disease. A similar trial in England found synovectomy of some benefit for the knee but not for metacarpophalangeal joints (7).

Chemical Synovectomy. Attempts to perform a "chemical synovectomy" by intra-articular injection of caustic substances to suppress synovitis have proved only partially successful. These agents have included sodium morrhuate, osmic acid, radioactive isotopes (yttrium 99, gold 198, and erbium 169), and two alkylating agents (nitrogen mustard and thiotepa). Experimental studies have shown that osmic acid can slow the growth of cartilage and epiphyseal bone. The results of thiotepa have been unpredictable, and the benefit of the alkylating agents and radioisotopes has not been established. These agents are not generally used in the United States except under research conditions.

Arthroplasty. Over the years, procedures for the reconstruction of joints have resulted in the greatest advances in the restoration of function in severely crippled joints. Rhea Barton (9) reported restored motion in an ankylosed hip with prevention of subsequent reunion by persistently repeated passive motion. He is credited with performing the first arthroplasty and producing an artificial pseudarthrosis. Subsequently, many successful operations of similar type were reported, but most of these joints eventually reankylosed. Many attempts were made to find a material to place over the denuded bony surface to prevent reunion. The nature and multiplicity of materials used for interposition were remarkable. Carnochan (19) of New York inserted a piece of wood between articulating surfaces of a resected temporomandibular joint; others tried flap of muscle, fascia lata, pig's bladder, and glass. In 1902 Jones covered the femoral head with a strip of gold foil in arthroplasty of the hip joint (73). He was able to report that effective motion was still present 21 years later. Also, in 1902 Murphy adopted the principle of interposing material for arthroplasties and used paraarticular fat and fascia lata in operations on the elbow, hip, knee, wrist, and shoulders (94).

Chromium-cobalt (Vitallium), as an interpositional metal, was introduced by Venable and Stuck in 1938 (160) and was first used by Smith-Peterson of Boston in 1939 (139) as an inert mold around which a fibrous tissue joint capsule was formed. In that same year Smith-Peterson reported excellent results in 29 hip arthroplasties and observed that this metal was well tolerated and solved the problem of breakage that had occurred with other materials. In the Smith-Peterson cup arthroplasty, the new metallic component is inserted in the acetabulum, and the femoral head remains as before except for surgical smoothing of the surface. In 1952 Moore of Columbia, South Carolina (92) and Thompson of New York (151) independently reported their experience with the reverse type of procedure in which the chromium-colbalt prosthesis replaced the femoral head and was inserted into the smoothed bony acetabulum. Both operations gave good results in the majority of patients and tended to have their devotees on a geographic basis, with the cup arthroplasty the choice among orthopedists trained in Boston and the Austin Moore or Thompson operations favored in New York.

The controversy about which was better soon came to an end with the introduction of the total joint replacement, which quickly made both of the other types of surgery obsolete in patients with arthritis. In this hip operation in which both the acetabular socket and the femoral head are replaced, both components may be metallic (89) or one metallic and the other a high-density polyethylene (21,22). The Charnley prostheses have essentially replaced the fully metallic ones because of their advantageously low index of friction. Although the total hip replacement was an English innovation, it was quickly adopted in the United States, and much of the development of the procedures for the hip and adaptation for operation on other joints have been American accomplishments.

The replacement of finger joints by prostheses began in the United States in the 1950s with the work of Flatt, who implanted metallic prostheses (43) and, subsequently, by Swanson and others working with prostheses molded of silicone (146). The implants proved helpful in overcoming deformities and improving hand function, especially in metacarpophalangeal joints and less so in the interphalangeal joints.

Great progress has also been made in the development of total knee replacement operations (Figure 11-3). Similar efforts are progressing rapidly for procedures applicable to wrists, elbows, shoulders, ankles, and feet.

It is appropriate to summarize this section by paying tribute to the role of the orthopedic surgeons over the years in the care of arthritis victims. The development of the total joint replacement is without question the single most important advance in the care of the arthritic patient crippled by severely damaged joints.

PSYCHOSOCIAL ASPECTS OF CARE

The psychosocial problems associated with arthritis surely must have troubled the first victim of that disability in prehistoric times. Imagine man unable to hunt to feed his family or to defend them. The woman could not care for their children or tend to her daily

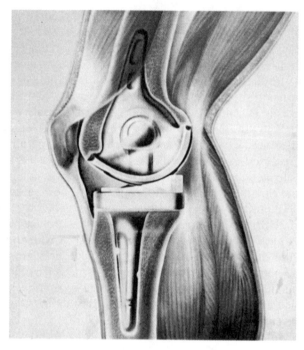

Figure 11-3. The January 1978 cover of *Scientific American* illustrating an artificial knee.

work, and neither could adequately meet the needs of the other. Then, as now, the arthritis patient was the victim of the cruel compound of pain, worries, and frustrations. In ancient and medieval times some segments of society, especially those with religious orientation, were concerned with the needs of the disabled. Though chiefly providing the basic needs for food and shelter, these benefactors with their deep religious convictions must have provided psychological support as well. With the development of hospitals in Europe, the need to help with the financial and other social requirements of the "sick poor" was recognized with the assignment of individuals, such as the almoners in England, to be responsible for helping to provide the necessary assistance.

Only in the present century, however, have community service organizations and hospitals gradually become conscious of the deep-seated psychological as well as social problems of disabled patients. Only in the past decade has such a formerly taboo subject as patients' sexual frustrations begun to be faced. With the recognition of the need of patients with arthritis for broad psychosocial support as well as physical, medical, and surgical care came the concept of the team approach in the provision of that care. As recounted in Chapter 9, recent decades have witnessed a steady growth of interest and training in rheumatologic aspects of their respective specialities among members of the various health professions. The common interest is well illustrated by the formation of the Arthritis Health Professions Association in 1965 and the fact that the two professional sections of the Arthritis Foundation, the ARA and the AHPA, hold joint annual and regional scientific meetings. This interest has brought together physical and occupational therapists, social workers, psychologists, and others working with physicians in caring for patients with rheumatic diseases.

ORGANIZATIONAL PROGRESS IN TREATMENT

Among the most important advances in the care of patients with rheumatic diseases have been those made possible by organizational developments. The increased awareness of the medical profession and the public of the importance of these diseases, the establishment of clinics and research centers, and the many other contributions of the American Rheumatism Association, the Arthritis Foundation, the Arthritis Health Professions Association, and the National Institute of Arthritis, Diabetes and Digestive and Kidney Diseases have been fundamental to the improved care of people with rheumatic diseases. These measures have been discussed in preceding chapters, and in this summary of progress in treatment it is necessary merely to emphasize the important part they have played.

REFERENCES

1. Allison W, Coonse GK: Synovectomy in chronic arthritis. Arch Surg 18:824-840, 1929
2. American Association for the Study and Control of Rheumatic Diseases. JAMA 103:1732-1734, 1801-1804, 1883-1884, 1934
3. American Heart Association, Rheumatic Fever Committee of the Council on Rheumatic Fever and Congenital Heart Disease: Preventing rheumatic fever. EM 113, 1972
4. Arthritis Foundation: Twentieth Anniversary Report, 1968
5. Arthritis Foundation Committee on the Evaluation of Synovectomy: Multicenter evaluation of synovectomy in the treatment of rheumatoid arthritis: report of results at the end of 3 years. Arthritis Rheum 20:765-771, 1977
6. Arthritis Health Professions Association: Rules of Procedure, revised January 1981
7. Arthritis and Rheumatism Council and British Orthopedic Association: A controlled trial of synovectomy of the knee and metacarpophalangeal joints in rheumatoid arthritis. Ann Rheum Dis 35:437-442, 1976
8. Atwater EC: Personal communication, 1983
9. Barton JR: On the treatment of ankylosis by the formation of artificial joints. North Am Med Surg J 3:279, 1827
10. Beck EG: Bismuth Paste in Chronic Supperations. St. Louis, CV Mosby, 1910
11. Bick EM: Source Book of Orthopedics. Second edition. New York, Hafner, 1965, p 330
12. Bigelow HJ: Resection of the head of the femur. Am J Med Sci 24:90, 1852
13. Billings F: Chronic focal infections and their etiologic relation to arthritis and nephritis. Arch Intern Med 9:484-498, 1912
14. Blumberg B, Bunim JJ, Calkins E, Pirani CL, Zvaifler NJ: ARA nomenclature and classification of arthritis and rheumatism (tentative). Arthritis Rheum 7:93-97, 1964
15. Boots RH, Miller CP: A study of neocinchophen in the treatment of rheumatic fever. JAMA 82:1928, 1924
16. Brewer EJ, et al: Criteria for the classification of juvenile rheumatoid arthritis. Bull Rheum Dis 23:712-719, 1972
17. Brewer EJ, et al: Revised criteria for the classification of juvenile rheumatoid arthritis. Arthritis Rheum 20(suppl):195-199, 1977
18. Bunim JJ, Pecket MM, Bollet AJ: Studies on metacostandralone and metacostandracin in rheumatoid arthritis. JAMA 157:311, 1955
19. Carnochan JM. In Bick EM: Sources of Orphopedics. Second edition. New York, Hafner, 1965
20. Cecil RL: Rheumatoid arthritis: a new method of approach to the disease. JAMA 100:1220-1227, 1933
21. Charnley J: Anchorage of the femoral head prosthesis to the shaft of the femur. J Bone Joint Surg 42B:28, 1960
22. Charnley J: Low Friction Arthroplasty of the Hip: Theory and Practice. Berlin, Springer-Verlag, 1979
23. Cheadle WB: Harvein lectures on the various manifestations of the rheumatic state as exemplified in childhood and early life. Lancet 1:821, 871, 921, 1889
24. Clark WS: Arthritis and Rheumatism: official journal of the American Rheumatism Association (editorial). Arthritis Rheum 1:1-3, 1958
25. Coburn AF: The Factor of Infection in the Rheumatic State. Baltimore, Williams & Wilkins, 1931
26. Coggeshall HC: Personal communication, 1984
27. Cohen AS, et al: Preliminary criteria for the classification of systemic lupus erythematosus. Bull Rheum Dis 21:643-648, 1971
28. A Conference on Rheumatic Diseases. JAMA 99:1020-1022, 1932
29. Cooperating Clinics Committee of the American Rheumatism Association: A controlled trial of cyclophosphamide in rheumatoid arthritis. N Engl J Med 283:883-889, 1970
30. Cooperating Clinics Committee of the American Rheumatism Association: A controlled trial of gold salt therapy in rheumatoid arthritis. Arthritis Rheum 16:353, 1973

31. Cupps TR, Fauci AS: The Vasculitides. Philadelphia, WB Saunders, 1981
32. Dawson MH, Boots RH: Recent studies in rheumatoid (chronic infectious, atrophic) arthritis. N Engl J Med 208:1030-1035, 1933
33. Decker J, et al: Dictionary of the Rheumatic Diseases. New York, Contact Associates, 1982
34. Diaz-Jimenez C, Lopez-Garcia E, Merchante A, Perianes J: The treatment of rheumatoid arthritis with nitrogen mustard. JAMA 147(15):1418-1419, 1951
35. Dilsen N, McEwen C, Poppel M, Gersh WJ, DiTata D, Carmel P: A comparative roentgenologic study of rheumatoid arthritis and rheumatoid (ankylosing) spondylitis. Arthritis Rheum 5:341-368, 1962
36. Domagk G: Beitrag zu Chemotherapie du bakteriellen Infectionen. Dtsch Med Wochenschr 6:250, 1935
37. Dreyer I, Reed CI: The treatment of arthritis with massive doses of vitamin D. Arch Phys Ther 16:537-540, 1935
38. Ellman P, Lawrence JS, Thorold GP: Gold therapy in rheumatoid arthritis. Br Med J 2:314-316, 1940
39. Empire Rheumatism Council Subcommittee: Gold therapy in rheumatoid arthritis: report of multi-centre controlled trial. Ann Rheum Dis 19:95-117, 1960
40. Empire Rheumatism Council Subcommittee: Gold therapy in rheumatoid arthritis: report of multi-centre controlled trial. Ann Rheum Dis 20:315-334, 1961
41. Faucher GJ: History of the Arthritis Foundation research fellowship program, 1951-1976. Arthritis Rheum 20(suppl):S249-S252, 1977
42. First Annual Report of the Director, National Institute of Arthritis, Diabetes, Digestive and Kidney Diseases. Washington, DC, Department of Health and Human Services, NIH Publication No. 82-2375, September 1982
43. Flatt AE: Care of the Arthritis Hand. St. Louis, CV Mosby, 1963
44. Fleming A: On the antibacterial action of cultures of penicillin, with special reference to their use in the isolation of B. influenzae. Br J Exp Pathol 10:226, 1929
45. Florey HW, Florey ME: General and local administration of penicillin. Lancet 1:387, 1943
46. Forestier J: L'aurotherapie dans les rhumatismes chroniques. Bull Mem Soc Med Hop Paris 53:323-327, 1929
47. Forestier J: Rheumatoid arthritis and its treatment by gold salts: results of 6 years experience. J Lab Clin Med 20:827, 1935
48. Fraser TN: Gold treatment in rheumatoid arthritis. Ann Rheum Dis 4:71-75, 1945
49. Fremont-Smith K, Bayles TB: Salicylate therapy in rheumatoid arthritis. JAMA 192:103, 1965
50. Freyberg RH, Baver JM: Vitamin D intoxication with metastatic calcification. University Michigan Hosp Bull 11-61, 1945
51. Freyberg RH, Block WD, Fromer MF: A study of sulfur metabolism and the effect of sulfur administration on chronic arthritis. J Clin Invest 19:423-435, 1940
52. Gall E: Address to the Board of Trustees and House of Delegates. Atlanta, Arthritis Foundation, 1983
53. Gall E: Professionalism Research and Directions: The AHPA in 1983. Presidential Address, Arthritis Health Professions Association, San Antonio, Texas, June 2, 1983
54. Garrod AB: The Nature and Treatment of Gout and Rheumatic Gout (Rheumatoid Arthritis). Third edition. London, Longmans Green & Co, Ltd, 1876
55. Goldthwait JE: Knee joint surgery for non-tuberculous conditions. Trans Am Orthoped Assoc 13:25, 1900
56. Gutman AB, Yü TF: Benemid as uricosuric agent in chronic gouty arthritis. Trans Assoc Am Physicians 64:279, 1951
57. Hapoienu BS, McDuffie FC: The Arthritis Foundation's research programs. Clin Rheumatol Pract 1:186-188, 1983
58. Hargraves MM, Richmond H, Morton R: Presentation of two bone marrow elements: the "tart cell" and the "L. E. cell." Proc Staff Meet Mayo Clin 23:23-28, 1948
59. Havens WP Jr: Clinical series. Internal medicine. Vol 3. Infectious Diseases and Internal Medicine. Chapter 18. Publication of the US Army Center of Military History. Washington DC, US Government Printing Office, 1968

60. Hench PS: A reminiscence of certain events before, during, and after the discovery of cortisone. Minn Med 36:705-710, 1953

61. Hench PS, Boland EW: The management of chronic arthritis and other rheumatic diseases among soldiers of the United States army. Ann Intern Med 24:808-825, 1946

62. Hench PS, Kendall EC, Slocumb CH, Polley HF: Effect of a hormone of the adrenal cortex (17 hydroxy-11 dehydrocorticosterone, Compound E) and of pituitary adrenocortico-tropic hormone on rheumatoid arthritis: preliminary report. Proc Staff Meet Mayo Clin 24:181, 1949

63. Hench PS, Kendall EC, Slocumb CH, Polley HF: The effect of cortisone and of ACTH on rheumatoid arthritis and rheumatic fever, Proceedings of Seventh International Congress on Rheumatic Diseases. Edited by Committee on Publications, American Rheumatism Association, Philadelphia, WB Saunders, 1952, pp 131-148

64. Hench PS, et al: The Present Status of the Problem of Rheumatism: a Review of Recent American and English Literature on "Rheumatism" and Arthritis. Ann Intern Med 8:1315-1374, 1495-1555, 1556-1580, 1935

65. Hench PS, et al: Rheumatism and arthritis: review of American and English literature for 1940 (Eighth Rheumatism Review). Ann Intern Med 15:1002, 1941

66. Hench PS, et al: Rheumatism and arthritis: a review of American and English literature of recent years (Ninth Rheumatism Review). Ann Intern Med 28:66, 1948

67. Hess EV, Fries JF, Klinenberg JR: A standard database for rheumatic disease. Arthritis Rheum 17:327-336, 1974

68. Hess EV, Fries JF, Klinenberg JR: A uniform database for rheumatic diseases. Arthritis Rheum 19:645-648, 1976

69. Hess EV, Fries JF, Klinenberg JR: A uniform database for rheumatic diseases. Arthritis Rheum 22:1029-1033, 1979

70. Hollander JL: Personal communication, 1984

71. Hollander JL, Brown BM Jr, Jessar RA, Brown CV: Hydrocortisone and cortisone injected into arthritic joints: comparative effects of, and use of, hydrocortisone as local anti-arthritic agent. JAMA 147:1629, 1951

72. Jaffe IA: Rheumatoid arthritis with arteritis. Ann Intern Med 61:556, 1964

73. Jones R, Lovett RW: Orthopedic Surgery. Baltimore, William Wood, 1929

74. Kracke RR, Parker FP: The etiology of granulopenia (agranulocytosis) with particular reference to the drugs containing the benzene ring. J Lab Clin Med 19:799, 1934

75. Kunkel HG, Tan EM: Autoantibodies and disease. Adv Immunol 4:351-395, 1964

76. Lamont-Havers R: Personal communication, 1982

77. Landé K: Die gunstige Beeinflüssung schleichender Dauerinfekte durch Solganal. Munchen Med Wochenschr 74:1132-1134, 1927

78. Libman E, Sacks B: A hitherto undescribed form of valvular and mitral endocarditis. Arch Intern Med 33:701-737, 1924

79. Lockie LM: Personal communication, 1984

80. MacLagan T: The treatment of acute rheumatism by salicin. Lancet I:342-343, 383-384, 1876

81. Mainland D, Sutcliffe MI: Hydroxychloroquine sulfate in rheumatoid arthritis: a 6 month double blind trial. Bull Rheum Dis 13:287-290, 1962

82. Malawista SE, Bensch KG: Human polymorphonuclear leukocytes: demonstration of microtubules and effect of colchicine. Science 156:521, 1967

83. Malawista SE, Bodel PT: The dissociation of colchicine of phagocytosis from increased oxygen consumption in human leukocytes. J Clin Invest 46:786, 1967

84. Masi AT, et al: Preliminary criteria for the classification of progressive systemic sclerosis (scleroderma). Arthritis Rheum 23:581-590, 1980

85. McCarty DJ: The American Rheumatism Association and the Arthritis Foundation: commentary on the 14 years of a happy union (editorial). Arthritis Rheum 22:1394-1395, 1979

86. McCarty DJ: Proceedings of the Conference on Pseudogout and Pyrophosphate Metabolism. Arthritis Rheum 19:2-3, 1976

87. McEwen C: Observations on rheumatology in the USSR. Arthritis Rheum 7:623-635, 1964

88. McEwen C, Ziff M, Carmel P, DiTata D, Tanner M: The relationship to rheumatoid arthritis of its so-called variants. Arthritis Rheum 1:481-496, 1958

89. McKee GK, Watson-Farrar J: Replacement of arthritic hips with McKee-Farrar prosthesis. J Bone Joint Surg 48B:245-259, 1966

90. Medsger TA Jr: Twenty-fifth Rheumatism Review. Arthritis Rheum 26:1983

91. Monell GC: Rheumatism: Acute and Chronic. New York, H C Langley, 1845

92. Moore AT: Metal hip joint: a new self locking Vitallium prosthesis. South Med J 45:1015, 1952

93. Muller W: Zu Frage der operativen Behandlung der Arthritis deformans und der chronischer Gelenkrheumatismus. Arch Forsch Klin Chir 47:1-39, 1894

94. Murphy JB: Arthroplasty. Am Surg 57:593, 1913

95. Murphy JB: Clinics of John B. Murphy. Vol 4, 1915

96. Murphy JB: Hypertrophic villous synovitis of the knee joint in synovial capsulectomy. Surg Clin Chicago 5:155-164, 1916

97. National Commission on Arthritis and Related Musculoskeletal Diseases: Arthritis Plan: Report to the Congress of the United States, April 1976. Washington DC, DHEW Publication No. 76-1150, 1976

98. Nichols EH, Richardson FL: Arthritis deformans. J Med Res 21:149-205, 1909

99. NIH Almanac 1981, US Department of Health and Human Services, NIH Publication No. 81-5, Bethesda, Maryland, Division of Public Information

100. Osler W: On the visceral complications of erythema exudativum multiforme. Am J Med Sci 110:629-649, 1895

101. Osler W: On the visceral manifestation of the erythema group of skin diseases. Trans Q Am Physicians 18:599-624, 1903

102. Osler W: The visceral lesions of the erythema group. Br J Dermatol 12:227-245, 1900

103. Outcome Standards for Rheumatology Nursing Practice, American Nurses Association, Division on Medical-Surgical Nursing Practice and Arthritis Health Professions Association. Atlanta, Arthritis Foundation, 1983

104. Page F: Treatment of lupus erythematosus with mepacrine. Lancet 2:755, 1951

105. Pemberton R: The control of rheumatism (editorial). JAMA 91:30-31, 1928

106. Pemberton R: History of the American Rheumatism Association. Prepared for the Seventh International Congress on Rheumatism, New York, 1949

107. Pemberton R, Foster GL: Studies on arthritis in the army, based on 400 cases. Arch Intern Med 25:243, 1920

108. Pemberton R, Robertson JW: Studies of arthritis in the army, based on 400 cases. I. Preamble and statistical analysis. Arch Intern Med 25:231-240, 1920

109. Pemberton R, Tompkins EH: Studies of arthritis in the army, based on 400 cases. II. Observations on the basal metabolism. Arch Intern Med 25:241-242, 1920

110. Pinals RS, et al: Preliminary criteria for the clinical remission of rheumatoid arthritis. Arthritis Rheum 24:1308-1315, 1981

111. Polley HF: Personal communication, 1984

112. Poole HM Jr: Introduction and welcome address: Conference Commemorating the 25th Anniversary of the Arthritis Foundation Research Fellowship Program. Arthritis Rheum 20(suppl):51-53, 1977

113. Proceedings of the Seventh International Congress on Rheumatic Diseases. Edited by Committee on Publications, American Rheumatism Association. Philadelphia, WB Saunders, 1952

114. Putnam CP: Salicylic acid in acute rheumatism. Boston Med Surg J 94:212, 1876

115. Rammelkamp CH, Denny FW, Wannamaker LW: Studies on the epidemiology of rheumatic fever in the armed services, in Rheumatic Fever. Edited by L Thomas. Minneapolis, University of Minnesota Press, 1952

116. Reuler JR, Girard DE, Nardone DA: The chronic pain syndrome: misconceptions and management. Ann Intern Med 93:588-596, 1980

117. Rheumatic Diseases. New York, Metropolitan Life Insurance Company, 1927

118. Riess L: Nachtrag zu innerlichen Anwendung der Salicylsäure, insbesonders bei dem acutem Gelenkrheumatismus. Berl Klin Wochenschr 13:86-89, 1876

119. Riess L: Uber die innerlichen Anwendung der Salicylsäure. Berl Klin Wochenschr 12:673-690, 1875

120. Riggs G: AHPA: past, present, future. Arthritis Rheum 25:704-705, 1982

References

121. Riggs G, Gall E, editors: Rheumatic Disease: Rehabilitation and Management. Boston, Butterworth Publishers, 1984
122. Robinson WD: Rheumatology as a subspecialty of internal medicine. Arthritis Rheum 11:262-266, 1968
123. Robitzek EH, Selikoss IJ, Ornstein GG: Chemotherapy of human tuberculosis with hydrazine derivative of isonicotinic acid. Q Bull Seaview Hosp 13:27, 1952
124. Rodnan GP: A brief history of the rheumatic diseases. Bull Rheum Dis 32:93-102, 1982
125. Rodnan GP: Growth and development of rheumatology in the United States: a bicentennial report. Arthritis Rheum 20:1149-1168, 1977
126. Rodnan GP, Benedek TG: The early history of antirheumatic drugs. Arthritis Rheum 13:145-165, 1970
127. Rodnan GP, Schumacher R: Primer on the Rheumatic Diseases. Eighth edition. Atlanta, Arthritis Foundation, 1983
128. Ropes MW, et al: Proposed diagnostic criteria for rheumatoid arthritis. Bull Rheum Dis 7:121-124, 1956
129. Ropes MW, et al: Revision of diagnostic criteria for rheumatoid arthritis. Bull Rheum Dis 9:175-176, 1958
130. Rose HM, Ragan C, Pearce E, et al: Differential agglutination of normal and sensitized sheep erythrocytes by sera of patients with rheumatoid arthritis. Proc Soc Exp Biol Med 68:1-6, 1948
131. Rundles RW, Wyngaarden JB, Hitchings GH, Elion GB, Silverman HR: Effects of a xanthine oxidase inhibitor on thiopurine metabolism, hyperuricemia, and gout. Trans Assoc Am Physicians 76:126, 1963
132. Rush B: Inquiries and observations. Philadelphia, Mathew Cary, 1805
133. Schantz A, Bugie E, Waksman SA: Streptomycin: a substance exhibiting antibiotic activity against gram-positive and gram-negative bacteria. Proc Exp Biol Med 55:66-69, 1944
134. Schottmüller H: Therpeutische Erfahrungen. Munch Med Wochenschr 74:861, 1927
135. Schüller M: Pathologie und Therapie der Gelenkentzündungen. Vienna, Urban & Schwartzberg, 1884
136. Schultz MP: The use of aminopyrine in rheumatic fever. Arch Intern Med 48:1138, 1931
137. Shen TY, et al: Non-steroid anti-inflammatory agents. J Am Chem Soc 85:488-489, 1963
138. Smith IW: Case of acute rheumatism treated with salicylic acid. Boston Med Surg J 94:511, 1876
139. Smith-Peterson MH: Arthroplasty of the hip: a new method. J Bone Joint Surg 21:269, 1939
140. Stecher RM: American Rheumatism Association: its origins, development and maturity. Arthritis Rheum 1:4-19, 1958
141. Stecher RM: Historical background of the Ligue International contre le Rhumatisme, Yearbook, Le Ligue International contre le Rhumatisme. Fourth edition, 1967
142. Steinbrocker O, Traeger CH, Batterman RC: Therapeutic criteria for rheumatoid arthritis. JAMA 140:659, 1949
143. Still GF: On a form of chronic joint disease in childhood. Med-Chir Trans 80:47-49, 1897
144. Stollerman GH: Rheumatic Fever and Streptococcal Infection. New York, Grune and Stratton, 1975
145. Stricker: Uber die Resultate der Behandlung der Polyarthritis rheumatica mit Salicylsäure. Berl Klin Wochneschr 1:15, 1876
146. Swanson AB: Silicone rubber implants for replacement of arthritis or destroyed joints in the hand. Surg Clin North Am 48:1113, 1968
147. Swett PP: Synovectomy in chronic infectious arthritis. J Bone Joint Surg 5:110-120, 1923
148. Swezey RI: Rational therapy and rehabilitation. Philadelphia, WB Saunders, 1978
149. Tan EM, et al: The 1982 revised criteria for the classification of systemic lupus erythematosus. Arthritis Rheum 1271-1277, 1982
150. Thomas A: Fact sheet for Tenth Anniversary of the Medical Council-Allied Health Professions Section, 1975
151. Thompson FR: Vitallium intermedullary hip prosthesis. NY J Med 52:3011, 1952
152. Todd EW: Antihaemolysin titres in haemolytic streptococcal infections and their significance in rheumatic fever. Br J Exp Pathol 13:248, 1932
153. Transactions, First Conference on Research and Education in the Rheumatic Diseases, 1953, Sponsored by the American Rheumatism Association, Arthritis and Rheumatism Foundation,

and the National Institute of Arthritis and Metabolic Diseases. New York, Arthritis Foundation, 1954

154. Transactions, Second Conference on Research and Education in the Rheumatic Diseases, 1957. New York, Arthritis Foundation, 1958

155. Tumulty PA, Harvey AM: The clinical course of disseminated lupus erythematosus: an evaluation of Osler's contributions. Bull Johns Hopkins Hosp 85:47-73, 1949

156. United Kingdom and United States Joint Report: The treatment of acute rheumatic fever in children: a cooperative clinical trial of ACTH, cortisone and aspirin. Circulation 11:343-377, 1955

157. United Kingdom and United States Joint Report: The treatment of acute rheumatic fever in children: a 5-year cooperative clinical trial of ACTH, cortisone and aspirin. Circulation 22:503-515, 1960

158. United Kingdom and United States Joint Report: The natural history of rheumatic fever and rheumatic heart disease: ten year report of a cooperative clinical evaluation of ACTH, cortisone, and aspirin. Circulation 32:457-476, 1965

159. van Breemen J: Le Ligue International contre le Rhumatisme: its origin and early years, Yearbook Le Ligue International contre le Rhumatisme. Second edition. 1955

160. Venable CS, Stuck WG: Electrolysis controlling factor in the use of metals in treating fractures. JAMA 111:1349, 1938

161. Vane JK: Inhibition of prostaglandin synthesis as a mechanism of action for aspirin-like drugs. Nature New Biol 234:231-238, 1971

162. Waine H, Baker F, Mettier SR: Controlled evaluation of gold therapy in rheumatoid arthritis. Calif Med J 66:295, 1947

163. Wallace SL, et al: Preliminary criteria for the classification of the acute arthritis of primary gout. Arthritis Rheum 20:895-900, 1930

164. What is Rheumatism? New York, Metropolitan Life Insurance Company, 1930

165. Whitman HH, Case DB, Laragh JH, Christian CL, Butstein G, Maricq H, LeRoy EC: Variable response to oral angiotensin-converting-enzyme blockade in hypertensive scleroderma patients. Arthritis Rheum 25:241-248, 1981

166. Wilson GM Jr, Huffman ER, Smyth CJ: Oral phenylbutazone in the treatment of acute gouty arthritis. Am J Med 21:232-236, 1956

Index

Index

Carlisle, James, 118
Case Western Reserve, early rheumatology, 9
Castle, William B., 111
Cecil, Russell L., 5, 8, 108
  Alphabet of Therapy for Rheumatoid Arthritis by, 123
  American Committee Against Rheumatism and, 23
  Arthritis and Rheumatism Foundation and, 38
  disease classification and, 73
  Medical Director, 79, 89
  Medical and Scientific Committee and, 43, 47
  presidential address, 34
  at senate hearings for NIAMD, 58
  vaccines for rheumatoid arthritis and, 123
Central Free Dispensary, early rheumatology, 9
Certificate of Incorporation of the Arthritis and Rheumatism Foundation, 79
Chapter Research Subcommittee, 86
Chapters, 44, 80, 81, 82, 91
Charcot's joints, 2, 74, 76
Charnley prostheses, 133
Chemical synovectomy, 132
Chemotherapeutic drugs for rheumatic diseases, 126
Chess, Leonard, 15
Chicago Rheumatism Society, 9
Children's Hospital in Los Angeles, 92
Chlorambucil, 126
Chloroform and joint resection, 132
Chloroquine for rheumatic diseases, 126
Christian, Charles L., 4, 15, 66, 67, 72
Chromium–cobalt in arthroplasty, 133
Chronic infectious arthritis, nomenclature, 73
Chrysotherapy in rheumatoid arthritis, 125
Cinchophen, 128
Clark, William S., 67, 81, 88, 95
Clarke, Clifford, 90, 92
Classical rheumatoid arthritis, diagnostic criteria, 77
Classification of rheumatic diseases, 27, 73, 115
Clay, Lucius, 51
Cleveland, Mather, 15
Cleveland City Hospital, 9
Clinical remission of rheumatoid arthritis, criteria, 77
Clinical Research Center, 85
Clinical Scholar, 84
Clinical seminars at ARA meetings, 62
Clinical Slide Collection on the Rheumatic Diseases, 69
Coates, V., 21
Codeine for rheumatic diseases, 129
Coggeshall, Howard C., 14, 18
Cohen, Alan S., 72
Colchicine discovery, 115, 121
Cole, Rufus, 15
Colloidal sulfur, 124
Colonic irrigations, 2
Columbia University, first rheumatology unit, 14
Committees
  on Affiliated Professional Sections, 100
  AHPA Research, 97
  ARA–AHPA coordination of, 96
  on Arthritis Advertising, 86
  Audiovisual Aids Subcommittee, 69

Committees (*Cont.*):
  for classification of rheumatic diseases, 73
  Cooperating Clinics, 78, 126
  on the Desirability and Feasibility of an American Journal on Arthritis and Rheumatism, 67
  Education, 69
  Education and Research, 37
  to evaluate synovectomy, 78
  Fellowship, 97
  Glossary, 75, 78
  Government Affairs, 91
  on Interrelationship with Arthritis and Rheumatism Foundation, 88
  Medical Advisory (MAC), 90
  Medical and Scientific, 90
  nomenclature and classification, 74
  Paramedical Section Education, 96
  Program–Project, 108
  Publication (ARA), 67
  Publications (AHPA), 97
  Research (AHPA), 97
  Rheumatology Subspecialty, 71
Compounds E and F, 118
Comroe, Bernard I., 16
Concept card, 26
Concurrent sessions at ARA meetings, 62
Conference proceedings, 69
Conference on rheumatic diseases, early, 27
Conference on rheumatic diseases of childhood, 92
Congress of the US, and arthritis programs, 84
Connective tissue disorders, 76, 121
Consulting Medical Directors of the Arthritis Foundation, 89
Cook County Hospital, 9
Cooperative Clinic Studies, 77
Copper bracelets, quackery campaign, 87
Cordery, Joy, 96, 97
Cornell Clinic, 4
Corticosteroids, 121, 127, 128
Cortisone
  discovery, 117, 118
  in inflammatory arthritis, 52
  NIAMD creation and, 58
  1949 paper on, 49
Coulter, John S., 32
Council on Pediatric Rheumatology, 92
Counseling services, 92
Councils, ARA, 73
Cowen, J. S., 59
Coyne, Nadene, 95
Crain, Darrell C., 18, 65
Cravener, Edward K., 11, 29
Croft, Jr., Joseph D., 69
Cummings, Nancy B., 109
Cyclo-oxygenase, aspirin inhibition, 128
Cyclophosphamide, 121, 126
Cytotoxic drugs, 126
Cytroen, George, 52

D

Database for rheumatic diseases, 78
Davidson, Harold M., 108
Davidson, Roland, 7